Nail Disorders: Practical Tips for Diagnosis and Treatment

Editor

ANTONELLA TOSTI

DERMATOLOGIC CLINICS

www.derm.theclinics.com

Consulting Editor
BRUCE H. THIERS

April 2015 • Volume 33 • Number 2

ELSEVIER

1600 John F. Kennedy Boulevard • Suite 1800 • Philadelphia, Pennsylvania, 19103-2899

http://www.theclinics.com

DERMATOLOGIC CLINICS Volume 33, Number 2
April 2015 ISSN 0733-8635, ISBN-13: 978-0-323-35973-3

Editor: Joanne Husovski
Developmental Editor: Susan Showalter

Dermatologic Clinics (ISSN 0733-8635) is published quarterly by Elsevier Inc., 360 Park Avenue South, New York, NY 10010-1710. Months of publication are January, April, July, and October. Business and editorial offices: 1600 John F. Kennedy Blvd., Suite 1800, Philadelphia, PA 19103-2899. Customer service office: 11830 Westline Drive, St. Louis, MO 63146. Periodicals postage paid at New York, NY, and additional mailing offices. Subscription prices are USD 365.00 per year for US individuals, USD 559.00 per year for US institutions, USD 425.00 per year for Canadian individuals, USD 681.00 per year for Canadian institutions, USD 495.00 per year for international individuals, USD 681.00 per year for international institutions, USD 165.00 per year for US students/residents, and USD 240.00 per year for Canadian and international students/residents. International air speed delivery is included in all *Clinics* subscription prices. All prices are subject to change without notice. **POSTMASTER:** Send address changes to *Dermatologic Clinics*, Elsevier Health Sciences Division, Subscription Customer Service, 3251 Riverport Lane, Maryland Heights, MO 63043. **Customer Service: 1-800-654-2452 (U.S. and Canada); 314-447-8871 (outside U.S. and Canada). Fax: 314-447-8029. E-mail: journalscustomerservice-usa@elsevier.com (for print support); journalsonlinesupport-usa@elsevier.com (for online support).**

Reprints. For copies of 100 or more, of articles in this publication, please contact the Commercial Reprints Department, Elsevier Inc., 360 Park Avenue South, New York, New York 10010-1710. Tel.: 212-633-3874; Fax: 212-633-3820; Email: repritns@elsevier.com.

The *Dermatologic Clinics* is covered in *MEDLINE/PubMed (Index Medicus)*, *Current Contents/Clinical Medicine*, *Excerpta Medica*, *Chemical Abstracts*, and *ISI/BIOMED*.

Contributors

CONSULTING EDITOR

BRUCE H. THIERS, MD
Professor and Chairman, Department of
Dermatology and Dermatologic Surgery,
Medical University of South Carolina,
Charleston, South Carolina

EDITOR

ANTONELLA TOSTI, MD
Professor of Clinical Dermatology, Department
of Dermatology and Cutaneous Surgery, Miller
School of Medicine, University of Miami,
Miami, Florida

AUTHORS

JOSETTE ANDRÉ, MD
Head, Dermatology Department, University
Hospitals Brugmann, St Pierre and Queen
Fabiola's Children Hospital, Université Libre de
Bruxelles, Brussels, Belgium

MARIE CAUCANAS, MD
Consultant, Dermatology Department,
University Hospitals Brugmann, St Pierre and
Queen Fabiola's Children Hospital, Université
Libre de Bruxelles, Brussels, Belgium

PATRICIA CHANG, MD, PhD
Dermatologist, Dermatology Service Social
Security General Hospital - IGSS, Guatemala
City, Guatemala

NILTON DI CHIACCHIO, MD, PhD
Dermatologic Clinic, Hospital do Servidor
Público Municipal de São Paulo, São Paulo,
Brazil

NILTON GIOIA DI CHIACCHIO, MD
Dermatologic Clinic, Hospital do Servidor
Público Municipal de São Paulo; Department of
Dermatology, Medical School of ABC, São
Paulo, Brazil

EMI DIKA, MD, PhD
Division of Dermatology, Department of
Experimental, Diagnostic and Specialty
Medicine, University of Bologna, Bologna,
Italy

JUDITH DOMÍNGUEZ-CHERIT, MD
Chief of Department of Dermatology, Insituto
Nacional de Ciencias Médicas y Nutrición
"Salvador Zubiran", México Distrito Federal,
Mexico

PIER ALESSANDRO FANTI, MD
Division of Dermatology, Department of
Experimental, Diagnostic and Specialty
Medicine, University of Bologna, Bologna,
Italy

DANIELA GUTIÉRREZ MENDOZA, MD
Professor of Dermatology, Department of
Dermatology, Hospital General "Dr Manuel
Gea González", México Distrito Federal,
Mexico

MATILDE IORIZZO, MD, PhD
Private Practice in Dermatology, Bellinzona,
Switzerland

NATHANIEL J. JELLINEK, MD
Dermatology Professionals, Inc, East
Greenwich, Rhode Island; Adjunct Assistant
Clinical Professor, Division of Dermatology,
University of Massachusetts Medical
School, Worcester, Massachusetts;
Assistant Clinical Professor, Department of
Dermatology, The Warren Alpert Medical
School at Brown University, Providence,
Rhode Island

**Dr. ESHINI PERERA, MBBS, B.MedSci,
MMed, MPH**
Department of Medicine, Dentistry and Health
Sciences, The University of Melbourne,
Parkville, Victoria; Department of Dermatology,
Epworth Hospital, Richmond, Victoria,
Australia

BIANCA MARIA PIRACCINI, MD, PhD
Associate Professor, Division of Dermatology,
Department of Experimental, Diagnostic and
Specialty Medicine, University of Bologna,
Bologna, Italy

ERICA REINIG, MD
Department of Pathology, Oregon Health
Sciences University, Portland, Oregon

PHOEBE RICH, MD
Department of Dermatology, Oregon Health
Sciences University, Portland, Oregon

BERTRAND RICHERT, MD, PhD
Clinical Professor, Dermatology Department,
University Hospitals Brugmann, St Pierre
and Queen Fabiola's Children Hospital,
Université Libre de Bruxelles, Brussels,
Belgium

ADAM I. RUBIN, MD
Assistant Professor of Dermatology,
Pediatrics, and Pathology and Laboratory
Medicine, Hospital of the University of
Pennsylvania; The Children's Hospital of
Philadelphia; Perelman School of Medicine at
the University of Pennsylvania, Philadelphia,
Pennsylvania

SAMANTHA L. SCHNEIDER, BA, MD
Department of Dermatology and Cutaneous
Surgery, University of Miami Miller School of
Medicine, Miami, Florida; Albert Einstein
College of Medicine, Bronx, New York

RODNEY SINCLAIR, MBBS, MD, FACD
Department of Medicine, Dentistry and
Health Sciences, The University of
Melbourne, Parkville, Victoria; Epworth
Hospital, Richmond, Victoria; Department
of Dermatology, Sinclair Dermatology, East
Melbourne, Victoria, Australia

SASHA STEPHEN, MD
Dermatology Resident, Department of
Dermatology, Hospital of the University of
Pennsylvania, Philadelphia, Pennsylvania

CURTIS T. THOMPSON, MD
Departments of Pathology, Dermatology, and
Biomedical Engineering, Oregon Health
Sciences University, Portland, Oregon

ANTONELLA TOSTI, MD
Professor of Clinical Dermatology, Department
of Dermatology and Cutaneous Surgery,
Miller School of Medicine, University of
Miami, Miami, Florida

NICOLE F. VÉLEZ, MD
Dermatology Professionals, Inc, East
Greenwich, Rhode Island

JONATHAN WEISS, MD
Chief Resident, Department of Dermatology
and Cutaneous Surgery, University of Miami
Miller School of Medicine, Miami, Florida

MARTIN N. ZAIAC, MD
Chairman, Department of Dermatology,
Herbert Wertheim College of Medicine, Florida
International University, Miami, Florida;
Director, Greater Miami Skin and Laser Center,
Mount Sinai Medical Center, Miami Beach,
Florida

Contents

Nail disorders are difficult to treat and often frustrating both for patients and clinicians. Because of the slow growth rate of the nail plate and the difficulty of getting the drug actives to penetrate the nail tissues, it is usually necessary to wait several months before seeing the results of treatments. This delay often leads to discontinuation of therapy by the patients. This article therefore helps clinicians to find the right treatment of the 5 most common nail disorders (brittle nails, onycholysis, paronychia, psoriasis, and onychomycosis) and provides practical tips that might improve patients' compliance.

The observation of a black-brown pigmentation of the nail is often alarming for the patient and for the clinician, as they are aware that it can be a possible clinical manifestation of melanoma of the nail apparatus. Luckily, however, nail melanoma is a much less frequent cause of brown-black nail color than other melanocytic and non-melanocytic pigmentations, which include subungual hematoma, exogenous pigmentations, and melanonychia due to benign conditions. A correct clinical history and careful examination help the clinician to distinguish the different conditions and to decide the correct management of melanonychia both in children and in adults.

This article reviews 6 nail disorders that, although easy to diagnose, are misdiagnosed frequently by dermatologists and general practitioners. Diagnostic clues are emphasized to familiarize readers with features that indicate the correct diagnosis. We focus on two common tumors (onychomatricoma and onychopapilloma), two rare genetic conditions that can be diagnosed owing to nail changes (Darier disease and nail patella syndrome), and two uncommon acquired disorders (the yellow nail syndrome and lichen striatus).

This article includes the etiology and pathophysiological data of each entity, classifying them as dermatologic, systemic, infectious, neoplastic, traumatic, and other classifications. The entities inherent to the periungual folds are also included, such as acute paronychia, chronic paronychia, retronychia, hangnails, hematomas of the proximal fold caused by oximeter, onychocryptosis, hypertrophy of the lateral folds, and infections caused by *Candida albicans, Pseudomonas,* and *Staphylococcus aureus.* Additionally, pathologies caused by diabetes mellitus, sepsis, endocarditis, drug reactions, and finally less frequent diseases that also affect the nail folds are discussed.

Diagnosing nail matrix diseases requires knowledge of the nail matrix function and anatomy. This allows recognition of the clinical manifestations and assessment of potential surgical risk. Nail signs depend on the location within the matrix (proximal or distal) and the intensity, duration, and extent of the insult. Proximal matrix involvement includes nail surface irregularities (longitudinal lines, transverse lines, roughness of the nail surface, pitting, and superficial brittleness), whereas distal matrix insult induces longitudinal or transverse chromonychia. Clinical signs are described and their main causes are listed to enable readers to diagnose matrix disease from the nail's clinical features.

Nails protect the fingertips and toes. Diseases affecting the nail can cause cosmetic disfigurement and social embarrassment. Physical functioning may be impaired. Disorders of the nail bed may cause pain or create difficulty grasping fine objects. The nail bed is the area beneath the nail plate between the lunula and the hyponychium. Disorders of the nail bed can cause onycholysis, subungual hyperkeratosis, and/or onychogryphosis. Ventral pterygium is less common. Tumors of the nail bed are rare and commonly missed.

 Videos of infiltrative anesthesia and nerve blockade of the bilateral dorsal/volar digital nerves accompany this article

Nail procedures require an effective and reliable approach to anesthesia of the distal digit. Several techniques have been described in the literature. Herein, the relevant anatomy of the nail unit, pain pathways, anesthetic options, and several injection approaches to achieve complete anesthesia are reviewed. Also considered are the potential pitfalls and complications and their management. Ultimately, the physician's approach must be individualized to the patient, procedure, and setting.

 A video of nail punch biopsy accompanies this article

Nail punch biopsy is used to obtain a tissue sample for the diagnosis and treatment of nail diseases. The best results will be possible if the surgeon is familiar with the anatomy and physiology of the nail apparatus. A punch biopsy can be used in all regions of the nail apparatus in the presence or absence of nail plate. When the procedure is performed with a careful handling of the anatomic site and specimen, in most cases a successful diagnosis can be achieved.

DERMATOLOGIC CLINICS

RELATED INTEREST

Nail and Skin Disorders of the Foot
Wesley W. Flint, Jarrett D. Cain, *Authors*
in
Managing and Treating Common Foot and Ankle Problems
John A. DiPreta, *Editor*
Medical Clinics of North America, March 2014, (Vol. 98, No. 2)

DOWNLOAD
Free App!

Review Articles
THE CLINICS

NOW AVAILABLE FOR YOUR iPhone and iPad

Preface

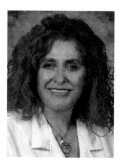

Antonella Tosti, MD
Editor

Nails are a difficult topic for many dermatologists, and training in nail disorders is often scarce. The purpose of this issue of *Dermatologic Clinics* is to make nail diseases easy to diagnose and treat. This will definitely improve the good care of patients.

Simple algorithms are proposed to approach treatment and management of most common disorders.

One article illustrates uncommon nail disorders that should not be missed, as their diagnosis is really easy.

Localization is another clue for diagnosis, and the use of this approach will allow expedited diagnosis for many conditions.

The article on nail surgery will teach, with the help of videos, how to perform simple procedures for diagnosis and treatment of most common nail disorders.

The final articles teach how to submit pathologic specimens and how nail clipping can be used beyond diagnosis of fungal infections.

I hope you will enjoy this issue and feel more confortable with your next patient with a nail disorder.

Antonella Tosti, MD
Department of Dermatology
and Cutaneous Surgery
Miller School of Medicine, University of Miami
1600 NW 10th Avenue, RMSB 2023A
Locator Code R-250
Miami, FL 33136, USA

E-mail address:
atosti@med.miami.edu

Dermatol Clin 33 (2015) ix
http://dx.doi.org/10.1016/j.det.2015.01.001
0733-8635/15/$ – see front matter © 2015 Published by Elsevier Inc.

Tips to Treat the 5 Most Common Nail Disorders

Brittle Nails, Onycholysis, Paronychia, Psoriasis, Onychomycosis

 CrossMark

Matilde Iorizzo, MD, PhD

KEYWORDS

- Treatment • Brittle nails • Onycholysis • Paronychia • Psoriasis • Onychomycosis

KEY POINTS

- Nail disorders are difficult to treat and often frustrating for both patients and clinicians.
- Knowledge of the disease to be treated and the patient's status are important for the choice of the best treatment option.
- The nail plate is a dead structure and clinicians cannot act on it. Treatment should be focused on the new growing nail.
- When facing a nail disorder, consider the presence of more than 1 disease at the same time (eg, psoriasis and onychomycosis/paronychia and onychomycosis/psoriasis and fragility).

INTRODUCTION

Nail disorders are difficult to treat and often frustrating for both patients and clinicians. Because of the slow growth rate of the nail plate (3 mm/mo for fingernails and 1.5 mm/mo for toenails) and the difficulty of getting the drug actives to penetrate the nail tissues, it is usually necessary to wait several months before seeing the results of treatments. This delay often leads to discontinuation of therapy by the patients.[1–3]

This article therefore helps clinicians (dermatologists and general practitioners) to find the right treatment of each of the 5 most common nail disorders and provides practical tips that might improve patients' compliance.

BRITTLE NAILS

Nail fragility is a condition that almost exclusively affects fingernails. It may be idiopathic or the consequence of factors that alter nail plate production and/or damage the already keratinized nail plate (trauma, dermatologic/systemic disorders, nutritional deficiencies, drug intake).[4]

Scanning electron microscopy studies indicate that idiopathic nail brittleness is associated with an intrinsic defect in the intercellular cement that holds together nail plate keratinocytes, with a disorganized protein and lipid structure and with a disorganized orientation of keratin filaments (in normal conditions, keratin filaments, rich in cysteine, a high-sulfur amino acid, are oriented parallel or perpendicular to the growth axis). This condition leads to nails that split, flake, and crumble, becoming soft and losing elasticity. In women, the intercellular keratinocyte bridges are constitutionally weaker than in men. Old age further weakens these bridges.[5,6] Environmental factors that produce progressive dehydration of the nail plate (eg, wet working conditions, minor trauma, and overaggressive manicuring) also

Disclosures: None.
Conflicts of interests: None.
Private Practice in Dermatology, Viale Stazione 16, Bellinzona 6500, Switzerland
E-mail address: matildeiorizzo@gmail.com

Dermatol Clin 33 (2015) 175–183
http://dx.doi.org/10.1016/j.det.2014.12.001
0733-8635/15/$ – see front matter © 2015 Elsevier Inc. All rights reserved.

play important roles in the development of nail brittleness.[7] However, some investigators disagree that nail plate cohesion is related to water content.[8]

When the amount of water in nails is reduced to less than 16%, they become brittle. Several factors are able to influence this water content, including lipids.[9] Normal nails contain 5% lipids, which are organized in a bilayer structure, parallel to the nail surface. Lipids fill certain ampullar dilatations of the dorsal plate and intercellular spaces in the ventral plate. Low lipid content decreases the nail's ability to retain water. A study showing a decrease in cholesterol sulfate in the nail plate with age, especially in women, suggests an important role of lipids in the development of nail brittleness in postmenopausal women.[6]

Nail fragility manifests with several nail plate abnormalities (onychoschizia, onychorrhexis, keratin granulation, erosions, distal wedge-shaped incision) that may be associated with the same nail or be present in different nails of the same patient.

Nail plate thinning caused by proximal nail matrix damage always involves the whole nail length and is often associated with abnormalities in the superficial nail plate. In contrast, damage to the distal matrix may produce alterations in the shape of the nail plate free edge.

Treatment

Nail fragility significantly impairs daily activities and occupational abilities. Its treatment requires time and patience (**Box 1**). Because the nail plate is a completely keratinized, dead structure, injuries cannot be repaired and each accident is added to the previous damage, rendering the nail plate more and more weak. The damaged portion is cured only when it grows out and is cut away.

Box 1
Treatment of brittle nails: key points

1. Reduce trauma and contact with water and detergents.
2. Wear cotton gloves under rubber gloves during manual work.
3. After any soaking, rehydrate nails with topical moisturizers.
4. Keep nails short and squared.
5. File nails in only one direction with a cardboard file.
6. Avoid nail cosmetics; they might be potentially harmful.
7. Remember that the keratin filaments are harder at a slightly acid pH.

If nail brittleness is caused by a dermatologic or a systemic condition, the first thing to do is to treat the disease to obtain an improvement of the symptom.

Oral supplementation with vitamins (especially biotin), oligoelements, and amino acids (especially cysteine) can be useful in improving nail strength.[10,11]

Biotin can be useful because it may improve the synthesis of the lipid molecules that produce binding between nail plate keratinocytes. The recommended oral dose is 5 to 10 mg/d, with 2 months being the average time before clinical improvements are observed. The recommended time of treatment is 3 to 6 months, but it is not clear how long the improvement in nail strength lasts after cessation of treatment.

Iron supplementation may be effective when serum ferritin levels are less than 10 ng/mL, but there are no studies showing that iron deficiency is strictly correlated with nail fragility. Zinc deficiency is known to cause soft and fragile nails, nail plate abnormalities, and chronic paronychia. Prolonged treatment with zinc 20 mg/d seems to improve brittle nails. Silica also seems to be important in improving the resistance of the nail plate through the cross-linking of keratins.[12,13]

Nail moisturizers are important in patients with brittle nails because of their occlusives, such as petrolatum or lanoline, and humectants, such as glycerin and propylene glycol. Alpha-hydroxy acids and urea may also be added to increase the water-binding capacity of the nail plate.[14]

Also available are lacquers specifically developed to restructure nails affected by dystrophy and fragility.[15,16]

A first lacquer owes its effectiveness to the presence of hydroxypropyl chitosan (HPCH), *Equisetum arvense*, and methylsulfonylmethane. When applied to the nails, HPCH forms a highly elastic, smooth, and almost invisible film that adheres to the nail structures, protecting them against physical injuries. HPCH is a chitosan derivative that has the advantage of being soluble in cold water without any pH correction, because the chitosan polymer backbone bears hydrophilic residues. These residues are thought to be the basis of the high affinity of HPCH with keratin. The presence of HPCH in the formulation is specifically effective in decreasing lamellar splitting.

A second lacquer made of 16% polyureaurethane, when applied to the nails, adheres tightly to the surface forming a strong but flexible waterproof barrier to environmental hazards. The active penetrates intercellular spaces and nail ridges, providing mechanical support.

Application of both lacquers is recommended once a day before bedtime.

Over-the-counter hardeners may instead paradoxically cause brittle nails if their use is prolonged. They increase the cross-link density over time, thus reducing the flexibility of the nail plate. When the nail plate is too rigid, it is also more prone to breaking and peeling. Moreover, because the hardeners are lacquers, they need to be periodically removed with a nail polish remover, which is a dehydrating agent.[14,17,18]

Artificial nails (sculptured acrylic nails, gel nails, nail mending kits, preformed plastic nails) are commonly used to cover and protect fragile nails but they can be responsible for fragility because of the materials used and the salon procedures used to apply these materials.[14,17,18]

ONYCHOLYSIS

Onycholysis means separation of the nail plate from the underlying nail bed caused by disruption of the onychocorneal band. It generally starts at the distal free margin of the nail plate and progresses proximally. Less often, it is the other way around. It may be idiopathic, traumatic, or secondary to nail bed disorders.[19–21]

Onycholysis is rarely associated with inflammation and the onycholytic area is usually smooth and whitish because of the presence of air under the detached nail plate. It may occasionally show a greenish or brown discoloration caused by colonization of the onycholytic space by chromogenic bacteria (*Pseudomonas aeruginosa*). Fungi are only secondary colonizers; treatment with systemic antifungals does not improve onycholysis, it just cures the sovrainfection.[19–21]

Treatment

The cornerstone of treatment is to minimize trauma to the affected digit and avoid as much as possible water/irritant environments. Nail bed disorders should always be ruled out first.[22] Then:

1. Clip away the onycholytic nail plate and repeat this procedure every 2 weeks until the nail plate grows attached.
2. The exposed nail bed should be carefully dried after each soaking.
3. Application of a topical antiseptic solution (2%–4% thymol in chloroform twice a day) on the exposed nail bed may be useful to prevent infections.
4. Sodium hypochlorite solution, 1 drop twice daily around the nail, removes *P aeruginosa* when present.

5. Avoid aggressive self-cleaning under the nail plate; this promotes the spreading of the detachment.
6. Do not confuse the skin debris collected under the nail plate with onychomycosis. Collect samples if necessary (evaluation of the affected area with the dermatoscope may help to rule out the presence of a fungus).[23]
7. Wear cotton gloves under rubber gloves during manual work.
8. Do not wear nail cosmetics and/or artificial nails until 3 months after the onycholysis has been resolved.

It is important to promote reattachment as soon as possible, otherwise the nail bed becomes cornified, producing dermatoglyphics like the tip of the digit (disappearing nail bed).[24] In this case the nail plate no longer adheres to the nail bed. It is generally assumed that the longer the disorder has been present, the less likely it is to resolve.

PARONYCHIA

Paronychia is an inflammatory disorder affecting proximal and lateral nail folds. A minor trauma (mechanical or chemical) usually breaks down the cuticle, the physical barrier between the nail plate and the nail folds, allowing the infiltration of infectious organisms, allergens, or irritants that cause an inflammatory reaction that impairs nail fold keratinization, preventing the formation of a new cuticle and maintaining the condition over time. Paronychia may occur in 2 forms: acute and chronic.

Acute Paronychia

The affected digit is painful, showing erythema, swelling, and sometimes pus discharge from the proximal and/or lateral nail folds. If the infection spreads to the nail bed, it may generate enough pressure to uplift the nail plate. Beau lines and onychomadesis may occur on the nail plate as a consequence of nail matrix damage.

Chronic Paronychia

The proximal and lateral nail folds show mild erythema and swelling. Beau lines and, less frequently, onychomadesis may occur. The nail plate sometimes presents a green discoloration of its lateral margins because of *P aeruginosa* colonization. Secondary colonization with *Candida albicans* and/or bacteria is also possible, causing self-limited episodes of painful acute inflammation. Depending on the major causal factor, chronic paronychia can be classified into several types.

Irritative reaction

This is the most common form of paronychia. The lesions are generally prominent with total involvement of the proximal nail fold. The condition worsens, especially if there is an underlying eczematous condition, such as atopic dermatitis. These patients have negative patch tests and negative provocative tests. They generally improve with preventive measures.

Contact allergy

Chronic paronychia is caused by an acute contact dermatitis of the proximal nail fold and the cause of sensitization may be disclosed by patch testing.

Food hypersensitivity

Patients complain of worsening of the periungual inflammation and itching immediately after handling raw food ingredients. The diagnosis can be made with a provocative test using fresh foods on the proximal nail fold (20-minute open patch test).

Candida hypersensitivity

Patients with chronic paronychia may develop a hypersensitivity to *Candida* antigens. These patients usually have an immediate reaction to the intradermal skin test to *Candida* antigens.

True Candida paronychia

This is very uncommon, except for patients with chronic mucocutaneous candidiasis and human immunodeficiency virus infection. Proximal nail fold inflammation is usually associated with proximal onycholysis or onychomycosis caused by *Candida*.

Treatment

Management of any form of paronychia always requires:

1. Avoidance of wet environments, chronic microtraumas, and contact with irritants or allergens (for at least 3 months after the condition is resolved).
2. Wearing cotton gloves under rubber gloves during manual work.
3. No aggressive/overzealous manicuring and nail cosmetics of any kind.
4. Treatment of the underlying predisposing condition as well as drug interruption if these are the causes.
5. Culture, radiographs, and/or biopsy, in recalcitrant cases, in order to exclude responsible disorders. They should always be ruled out when only 1 digit is involved.

Specifically, acute paronychia requires:

1. Drainage of the abscess, if present, and local medications with antiseptics (2%–4% thymol in chloroform twice a day) to obtain relief of inflammation and pain.
2. Sodium hypochlorite solution 1 drop twice daily around the nail to remove *P aeruginosa* when present.
3. A topical combination of fusidic acid and betamethasone 17-valerate cream applied twice a day.[25] This combination reduces pain first, then inflammation and swelling.
4. Mupirocin cream in the morning and clobetasol cream in the evening is an alternative option.

Chronic paronychia instead requires:

1. Application of a mild-potency topical steroid (methylprednisolone aceponate 0.1% cream) at bedtime.[26]
2. Tacrolimus 0.1% ointment applied twice a day as an alternative.[27]
3. A cream containing piroctone olamine and climbazole, applied twice a day for 3 months.[28] This product combines antiinflammatory, antimicrobial, and protective activities. Patients using this cream showed disappearance of the inflammatory signs and growth of a normal nail plate, smooth and shiny. Complete cuticle regrowth was seen in greater than 50% of cases.
4. Systemic steroids (methylprednisone 20 mg/kg/d) for few days in severe cases, when several digits are affected.
5. Triamcinolone acetonide 2.5 mg/mL into affected nail folds (monthly injections) as an alternative in severe cases. Topical lidocaine can be applied 1 hour before the injections to reduce pain.

Systemic antifungals are often useless because chronic paronychia is not a mycotic infection. *Candida* is just a colonizer of the proximal nail fold that disappears when the proximal nail fold barrier is restored.[26]

PSORIASIS

Nail changes are reported in up to 50% of psoriatic patients and they might be the only manifestation of the disease. Several nails are usually affected. Depending on the anatomic area affected, the disease presents with different signs: irregular pitting, surface ridging, and nail plate thickening for psoriasis of the nail matrix; salmon patches, onycholysis with erythematous border splinter hemorrhages, and subungual hyperkeratosis for psoriasis of the nail bed. All these signs could present together in the same patient and even in the same nail.[29]

The impact on quality of life of this disorder is very high and the need for effective treatments should be met as soon as possible. There are many treatments currently under clinical trials for psoriasis: the difficulty is to find an agent effective for nail psoriasis with absent or minimal systemic side effects. The research on psoriasis should probably be focused on new vehicles for old drugs rather than new actives.

Treatment

At present there is no cure for psoriasis. Available treatments require time and patience and, in most cases, the results are scarce. It is important to remind patients that nail psoriasis is often worsened by mechanical trauma (Koebner phenomenon). It is also scarcely influenced by sun exposure and other environmental factors that improve skin psoriasis.

Reassuring the patient is generally the best treatment option for mild nail psoriasis. No treatment or mild emollients/lacquers containing urea might be an option.

For more severe cases, application of a cream containing calcipotriol and betamethasone dipropionate at bedtime is useful, especially for nail bed psoriasis.[30,31] The effectiveness can be improved applying the product directly on the nail bed, with an overnight occlusion, after trimming the detached nail plate. This treatment is easily accepted by patients, even though recurrences are frequent after discontinuation. Application of topical tazarotene 0.1%, with or without occlusion, is another good option. Irritation of the nail folds is a frequent side effect.[32,33]

Subungual hyperkeratosis and nail thickening respond better than onycholysis and pitting.

Both calcipotriol and tazarotene are unable to reach the nail matrix if applied on the proximal nail fold and they are almost useless for nail matrix psoriasis. In nail matrix psoriasis, high-potency steroids, such as clobetasol propionate 0.05% cream, are a better option even though it has been proved that, if applied for long periods, they may cause acroatrophy (disappearing digit syndrome).[34]

When few digits are affected, triamcinolone acetonide 10 mg/mL (maximum 4 injections of 0.1 mL per digit) could be injected into the proximal nail fold (in patients with nail matrix psoriasis) or in the lateral nail folds (in patients with nail bed psoriasis).[35] Injections should be repeated monthly for 6 months, then every 6 weeks for the next 6 months, and then every 2 months for 6 to 12 months. Side effects include hemorrhages, pigmentary changes, and skin atrophy. Benefits should be apparent in 2 to 3 months. Subungual hyperkeratosis and nail thickening respond better than onycholysis and pitting. However, for improving pitting this is the best option.

Local anesthesia with ethyl chloride or topical lidocaine is generally necessary to make the treatment less painful. To reduce pain, needle-free jet injectors are also available, although they may cause more side effects. The steroid can also be mixed with a local anesthetic (this must not include epinephrine). An anesthetic block might be necessary to treat nail bed psoriasis.

Oral acitretin 0.3 mg/kg/d for at least 6 months is a good treatment of severe nail matrix and nail bed psoriasis.[36] The dosage can be increased to 0.5 to 0.75 mg/kg/d, but with more side effects. Subungual hyperkeratosis and thickening improve better than onycholysis and pitting. If the nail plate is thin and fragile, it is better not to use acitretin because it could worsen the condition.

Subcutaneous methotrexate (15 mg per week) and a low dosage of oral cyclosporin (2.5 mg/kg/d) have also been used with success.[37,38] The former seems to give better results for nail matrix psoriasis, the latter for nail bed psoriasis.

Biologic agents (adalimumab, etanercept, infliximab, ustekinumab) have enriched the therapeutic armamentarium against psoriatic nails, but they are generally restricted to patients with a concomitant skin and/or joint psoriasis because of their high costs and toxicity. However, a consensus on the use of these drugs for nail psoriasis is still lacking (**Table 1**).[39]

ONYCHOMYCOSIS

Onychomycosis means the invasion of the nail by fungi (dermatophytes, molds, yeasts). Different clinical patterns of infection are described, depending on the way and the extent by which fungi colonize the nail. The type of nail invasion depends on both the fungus responsible and host susceptibility. Onychomycosis is an infection and should always be treated.

Treatment

Treatment of onychomycosis is usually time consuming and requires considerable patience, because of the slow growth rate of the nail plate and the difficulty of getting actives to reach the infected area.

The choice of the best therapeutic approach is based on numerous factors that should always be established before starting any treatment:

Table 1
Treatment of nail psoriasis depending on the affected site

Nail Matrix Psoriasis	Nail Bed Psoriasis
Clobetasol propionate 0.05% cream (1/d UO)	Calcipotriol/betamethasone cream (1/d UO)
Triamcinolone acetonide 10 mg/mL (4 × 0.1-mL IL injections)	Tazarotene 0.1% cream or ointment (1/d UO)
	Clobetasol propionate 0.05% cream (1/d UO)
Acitretin 0.3 mg/kg/d (OA)	Triamcinolone acetonide 10 mg/mL (4 × 0.1-mL IL injections)
Methotrexate 15 mg/wk (SC)	
Biologics	Acitretin 0.3 mg/kg/d (OA)
	Cyclosporine 2.5 mg/kg/d (OA)
	Biologics

Abbreviations: IL, intralesional; OA, oral administration; SC, subcutis; UO, under occlusion.

---

patient's age and health, responsible fungus, clinical type of onychomycosis, number of affected nails, and severity of nail involvement. The concomitant presence of tinea pedis (and tinea capitis in children) should always be ruled out.[40]

The goal of antifungal therapy should be mycological cure, obtained when both microscopic and cultural examinations are negative. To assess clinical cure, patients should be followed for at least 6 months after discontinuation of treatment. Recurrences and reinfections are always possible.

There are currently 3 main strategies to treat onychomycosis: oral therapies, topical therapies, and a combination of both.[41] Oral treatments are much more effective than topical ones, but they are also associated with more systemic side effects and drug interactions. Topicals cause fewer side effects but their poor nail penetration limits their efficacy. For this reason, clinical studies are trying to find better penetration enhancers as well as new actives.

Topical monotherapy is usually recommended for:

- Distal subungual onychomycosis (DSO) affecting less than 50% of the nail without matrix involvement, without yellow streaks along the lateral margin of the nail, and without yellow onycholytic areas in the central portion of the nail (dermatophytoma).
- White superficial onychomycosis (WSO) in the classic form
- Onychomycosis caused by molds (except for those caused by *Aspergillus* sp)
- Patients unwilling or unable to tolerate oral therapy
- Patients requiring maintenance therapy after a course of oral therapy

Oral monotherapy is more suitable for:

- DSO affecting greater than 50% of the nail, including matrix

- DSO affecting more than 2 nails
- Proximal subungual onychomycosis
- WSO in their deep form
- Patients not responding after 6 months of topical monotherapy alone

Penetration of a topical antifungal through the nail plate requires a vehicle that is specifically formulated for transungual delivery. Two vehicles are currently available:

1. Water-insoluble polymers that create a film on the nail surface. Daily or weekly application and removal with organic solvents is required; nail filing is also necessary to reduce nail thickness, thus allowing better penetration of the actives.
2. Hydroalcoholic solutions of HPCH forming an invisible non-irritating film that is easily removable with water.

Topical agents well known to be effective against onychomycosis are amorolfine 5%, a morpholine derivative with a broad-spectrum fungicidal and fungistatic activity, and ciclopirox olamine 8%, a hydroxypyridone derivative with a broad-spectrum fungicidal and sporicidal activity.

Amorolfine nail lacquer should be applied twice per week for 6 to 12 months. Adverse events are rare (<5%) and include burning, itching, redness, and pain near the application site. In the literature, randomized controlled trials evaluating the efficacy and safety of this agent are scarce. Moreover, it is more cost-effective than ciclopirox olamine 8% nail lacquer.

Ciclopirox olamine nail lacquer should be applied daily for 6 to 12 months. Adverse events are rare (<1%) and include burning, itching, and redness near the application site. It is widely used in children with successful outcomes.[42] In a multicentre, randomized, 3-arm, placebo-controlled, parallel groups, evaluator-blinded study, ciclopirox olamine 8% in hydroalcoholic solution of HPCH showed superior properties in terms of affinity to keratin, nail permeation, and easiness to use compared with the vinyl resin–based lacquer.[43]

Recently, 2 new agents have been approved by the US Food and Drug Administration for the topical treatment of onychomycosis: efinaconazole and tavaborole.

Efinaconazole 10%, a triazole with a broad-spectrum antifungal activity, has been released on the market to treat DSO caused by dermatophytes in adults.[44] It presents as a solution that has to be applied daily for 9 to 12 months. No periodic removal is required. Its low affinity for keratin results in very good nail penetration. Adverse events are rare (comparable with vehicle) and include mild site dermatitis and vesicles.

Tavaborole 5% is an oxaborole, also with a broad-spectrum antifungal activity, and was released to treat onychomycosis caused by dermatophytes in adults.[45] It is a solution that should be applied daily for 12 months to the entire nail surface and under the tip of the plate. The degree of penetration through the nail plate has been shown to be superior to ciclopirox. Adverse events include application site exfoliation and erythema.

The cure rate of onychomycosis treated with topicals can be improved by mechanical or chemical avulsion of the affected nail plate in order to enhance penetration of the actives. Microporation (drilling of small holes), phonophoresis (low-frequency ultrasonography), or the use of 40% urea–based preparations have been found to enhance drug permeation through the nail plate. Chemical enhancers are usually more practical than physical enhancers; they are cheaper and more easy to use (they are placed on the affected nail, under occlusion, for 1 week maximum). With this technique, topical antifungals otherwise ineffective to treat onychomycosis, can be used with success. For example, terbinafine cream, applied twice a day and preferably under occlusion, is a good option.

Among systemic treatments, terbinafine has been proved to be more effective than other agents such as itraconazole, fluconazole, or griseofulvin and is, therefore, considered the first-line treatment. Percentages of cure rates obtained with systemic drugs vary from study to study.[41]

Terbinafine is an allylamine with a fungistatic and fungicidal effect. Following oral administration, terbinafine is rapidly absorbed and widely distributed to body tissues including the nail matrix. Nail terbinafine concentrations are detected within 1 week after starting therapy and persist for at least 30 weeks after the completion of treatment. Terbinafine can be administered at the continuous dosage of 250 mg daily or as pulse therapy (also called intermittent) at the dosage of 500 mg daily (250 mg × 2) for 1 week a month. Treatment duration is at least 6 weeks for fingernails and 12 weeks for toenails. Dosages in children are: less than 20 kg, 62.5 mg/d; 20 to 40 kg, 125 mg/d; more than 40 kg, 250 mg/d. Terbinafine is available in tablets or granules.

Interactions with other drugs are rare, even though terbinafine is a competitive inhibitor of the cytochrome P450–linked enzyme 2D6. Terbinafine is usually well tolerated and mild adverse events involve the gastrointestinal system. Taste alterations (metallic taste) typically occur 5 to 8 weeks after starting treatment. Skin rashes are common and are sometimes severe. Terbinafine is not recommended in patients with liver disorders but it is safe for diabetic patients. It can be used for patients with celiac disease but the formulation is not lactose free.

Itraconazole is a synthetic triazole, fungistatic and with a much broader spectrum of action. For this reason it has shown more efficacy in mixed infections and Candida onychomycosis. Itraconazole can be detected in nails 1 week (fingernails) to 2 weeks (toenails) after the start of therapy and it is still detectable in nails 27 weeks after stopping administration, which is why it is administered with a pulse therapy, at the dosage of 200 to 400 mg daily for 1 week a month. Treatment duration is at least 6 weeks for fingernails and 12 weeks for toenails. Dosages in children are 5 mg/kg/d pulsed (2 pulses for fingernails and 3 pulses for toenails). Itraconazole is available in tablets or oral suspension.

This drug should be administered with a high-fat meal and/or acidic beverage to improve its absorption (the suspension needs an empty stomach). Agents that increase gastric alkalinity reduce itraconazole absorption. If there are no therapeutic alternatives, itraconazole should be administered 2 hours before one of these agents.

With itraconazole, the basis of drug interactions is the inhibition/induction of the cytochrome P450–linked enzyme 3A4. Care must be taken with elderly people taking multiple drugs. Adverse effects may involve the gastrointestinal system, the liver, and the skin. Its use has also been associated with congestive heart failure. Itraconazole is safe for patients with celiac disease and is lactose free.

In patients with poor prognostic factors suggesting possible treatment failure, options are[46]:

- Combination therapy: association of a systemic treatment and a topical treatment, with the latter to be continuously applied even when onychomycosis is cured, for at least 6 months.

- Supplemental therapy with terbinafine or itraconazole: the suggested regimen is 250 mg/d of continuous terbinafine or itraconazole 400 mg/d for 1 week a month. At month 6, if the culture is still positive and/or onychomycosis has progressed proximally, the patient can have an extra month of the drug.
- Sequential therapy with itraconazole followed by terbinafine: the suggested regimen is 2 pulses of itraconazole 400 mg/d for 1 week a month followed by 1 to 2 pulses of terbinafine 500 mg/d for 1 week a month. One pulse is usually given for fingernail onychomycosis and 2 pulses for toenail onychomycosis.
- Consider an alternative approach such as photodynamic therapy (PDT) or lasers:
  1. PDT: after chemical avulsion of the nail plate, a 5-aminolevulinic acid cream is applied under occlusion for 3 hours, then removed and the nail area irradiated for 8 minutes, with a light-emitting diode lamp (red light with a narrow spectrum at 630 nm). The light dose to be used is 37 J/cm^2 and the lamp should be placed 50 to 80 mm from the skin. One treatment is usually not effective and other irradiations, at intervals of 15 to 21 days, are necessary. The optimal light source and the number of PDT treatments that are necessary to cure all onychomycosis remain to be established.
  2. Lasers: the affected nail is irradiated with a laser beam whose wavelength is absorbed by the fungus. The absorbed energy is converted into heat and the increased temperature kills the pathogen without damaging the surrounding tissues (the chromophore is present only in the pathogen). Lasers have been approved in many countries to treat onychomycosis but they are still under investigation to find the best laser and treatment parameters for each situation. Comparing lasers is not easy and single treatments are expensive. They can be considered an alternative approach to treating onychomycosis but they are far from achieving the cure rates obtained with drugs.

REFERENCES

1. Baran R, deBerker D, Holzberg M, et al, editors. Baran and Dawber's diseases of the nails and their management. 4th edition. Oxford (UK): Wiley Blackwell; 2012.
2. Piraccini BM, Iorizzo M, Antonucci A, et al. Treatment of nail disorders. Therapy 2004;1:159–67.
3. Shemer A, Daniel CR III. Common nail disorders. Clin Dermatol 2013;31:578–86.
4. Iorizzo M, Pazzaglia M, Piraccini BM, et al. Brittle nails. J Cosmet Dermatol 2004;3:138–44.
5. Helmdach M, Thielitz A, Ropke EM, et al. Age and sex variation in lipid composition of human fingernail plates. Skin Pharmacol Appl Skin Physiol 2000;13:111–9.
6. Brosche T, Dressler S, Platt D. Age-associated changes in integral cholesterol and cholesterol sulfate concentrations in human scalp hair and finger nail clippings. Aging 2001;13:131–8.
7. Lubach D, Beckers P. Wet working conditions increase brittleness of nails, but do not cause it. Dermatology 1992;185:120–2.
8. Duarte AF, Correia O, Baran R. Nail plate cohesion seems to be water independent. Int J Dermatol 2009;48:193–5.
9. Stern DK, Diamantis S, Smith E, et al. Water content and other aspects of brittle versus normal fingernails. J Am Acad Dermatol 2007;57:31–6.
10. Colombo VE, Gerber F, Bronhofer M, et al. Treatment of brittle fingernails and onychoschizia with biotin: scanning electron microscopy. J Am Acad Dermatol 1990;23:1127–32.
11. Hochman LG, Scher RK, Meyerson MS. Brittle nails: response to daily biotin supplementation. Cutis 1993;51:303–5.
12. Scheinfeld N, Dahdah MJ, Scher R. Vitamins and minerals: their role in nail health and disease. J Drugs Dermatol 2007;6:782–7.
13. Haneke E. Onychocosmeceuticals. J Cosmet Dermatol 2006;5:95–100.
14. Iorizzo M, Piraccini BM, Tosti A. Nail cosmetics in nail disorders. J Cosmet Dermatol 2007;1:53–8.
15. Sparavigna A, Caserini M, Tenconi B, et al. Effects of a novel nail lacquer based on hydroxypropyl-chitosan (HPCH) in subjects with fingernail onychoschizia. J Dermatolog Clin Res 2014;2:1013–7.
16. Available at: www.nuvail-rx.com. Accessed May, 2014.
17. Baran R, André J. Side effects of nail cosmetics. J Cosmet Dermatol 2005;4:204–9.
18. Dahdah MJ, Scher R. Nail diseases related to nail cosmetics. Dermatol Clin 2006;24:233–9.
19. Baran R, Badillet G. Primary onycholysis of the big toenails: a review of 113 cases. Br J Dermatol 1982;106:529–34.
20. Daniel CR III, Iorizzo M, Piraccini BM, et al. Simple onycholysis. Cutis 2011;87:226–8.
21. Daniel CR III, Daniel MP, Daniel CM, et al. Chronic paronychia and onycholysis: a 13 year experience. Cutis 1996;58:397–401.
22. Kechijian P. Onycholysis of the fingernails: evaluation and management. J Am Acad Dermatol 1985;12:552–60.

23. Piraccini BM, Balestri R, Starace M, et al. Nail digital dermoscopy (onychoscopy) in the diagnosis of onychomycosis. J Eur Acad Dermatol Venereol 2013;27:509–13.

24. Daniel CR III, Tosti A, Iorizzo M, et al. The disappearing nail bed: a possible outcome of onycholysis. Cutis 2005;76:325–7.

25. Wollina U. Acute paronychia: comparative treatment with topical antibiotic alone or in combination with corticosteroid. J Eur Acad Dermatol Venereol 2001; 15:82–4.

26. Tosti A, Piraccini BM, Ghetti E, et al. Topical steroids versus systemic antifungals in the treatment of chronic paronychia: an open, randomized double-blind and double dummy study. J Am Acad Dermatol 2002;47:73–6.

27. Rigopoulos D, Gregoriou S, Belyayeva E, et al. Efficacy and safety of tacrolimus ointment 0.1% vs. betamethasone 17-valerate 0.1% in the treatment of chronic paronychia: an unblinded randomized study. Br J Dermatol 2009;160:858–60.

28. Piraccini BM, Bruni F, Alessandrini A, et al. Ecocel Plus Cream: combination of anti-inflammatory, anti-microbial and sealing effects in the treatment of fingernail chronic paronychia: clinical study on 18 cases. Esperienze Dermatologiche 2014;16:29–33.

29. Edwards F, de Berker D. Nail psoriasis: clinical presentation and best practice recommendations. Drugs 2009;69:2351–61.

30. Tosti A, Piraccini BM, Cameli N, et al. Calcipotriol ointment in nail psoriasis: a controlled double blind comparison with betamethasone dipropionate and salicylic acid. Br J Dermatol 1998;139:655–9.

31. Tzung TY, Chen CY, Yang CY. Calcipotriol used as monotherapy or combination therapy with betamethasone dipropionate in the treatment of nail psoriasis. Acta Derm Venereol 2008;88:279–80.

32. Rigopoulos D, Gregoriou S, Katsambas A. Treatment of psoriatic nails with tazarotene cream 0.1% vs clobetasol propionate 0.05% cream: a double-blind study. Acta Derm Venereol 2007;87:167–8.

33. Fischer-Levancini C, Sánchez-Regaña M, Llambí F, et al. Nail psoriasis: treatment with tazarotene 0.1% hydrophilic ointment. Actas Dermosifiliogr 2012; 103:725–8.

34. Wolf R, Tur E, Brenner S. Corticosteroid-induced "disappearing digit". Arch Dermatol 1990;23:755–6.

35. de Berker DA, Lawrence CM. A simplified protocol of steroid injection for psoriatic nail dystrophy. Br J Dermatol 1998;138:90–5.

36. Tosti A, Ricotti C, Romanelli P, et al. Evaluation of the efficacy of acitretin therapy for nail psoriasis. Arch Dermatol 2009;145:269–71.

37. Mahrle G, Schulze HJ, Farber L, et al. Low dose short term cyclosporine versus etretinate in psoriasis: improvement of skin, nail and joint involvement. J Am Acad Dermatol 1995;32:78–88.

38. Gumusel M, Ozdemir M, Mevlitoglu I, et al. Evaluation of the efficacy of methotrexate and cyclosporine therapies on psoriatic nails: a one-blind, randomized study. J Eur Acad Dermatol Venereol 2011;9:1080–4.

39. Kyriakou A, Patsatsi A, Sotiriadis D. Biologic agents in nail psoriasis: efficacy data and considerations. Expert Opin Biol Ther 2013;13:1707–14.

40. Baran R, Hay RJ, Garduno JI. Review of antifungal therapy, part II: treatment rationale, including specific patient population. J Dermatolog Treat 2008; 19:168–75.

41. Iorizzo M, Piraccini BM, Tosti A. Today's treatment option for onychomycosis. JDDG 2010;8:875–9.

42. Fallon Friedlander S, Chau YC, Chau YH, et al. Onychomycosis does not always require systemic treatment for cure: a trial using topical therapy. Pediatr Dermatoe 2013;3:316–22.

43. Baran R, Tosti A, Hartmane I, et al. An innovative water-soluble biopolymer improves efficacy of ciclopirox nail lacquer in the management of onychomycosis. J Eur Acad Dermatol Venereol 2009;23:773–81.

44. Elewski BE, Rich P, Pollak R, et al. Efinaconazole 10% solution in the treatment of toenail onychomycosis: two phase III multicenter, randomized, double-blind studies. J Am Acad Dermatol 2013; 68:600–8.

45. Elewski BE, Tosti A. Tavaborole for the treatment of onychomycosis. Expert Opin Pharmacother 2014; 10:1439–48.

46. Gupta AK, Paquet M. Improved efficacy in onychomycosis treatment. Clin Dermatol 2013;31:555–63.

Tips for Diagnosis and Treatment of Nail Pigmentation with Practical Algorithm

Bianca Maria Piraccini, MD, PhD*, Emi Dika, MD, PhD,
Pier Alessandro Fanti, MD

KEYWORDS

- Nail pigmentation • Melanonychia • Melanoma • Nevus • Melanocytes • Dermoscopy

KEY POINTS

- A brown pigmentation of the nail is not necessarily due to melanin.
- Dermoscopy should be used routinely when dealing with nail pigmentations.
- Clinical history, number of nails involved, and associated nail and internal diseases are important parameters to consider when evaluating melanic nail pigmentation.
- Childhood longitudinal melanonychia of a single digit is most commonly a nevus.
- Adult-onset melanonychia of a single digit should be carefully evaluated and often needs a bioptic examination.

The observation of a black-brown pigmentation of the nail is often alarming for the patient and for the clinician, as they are aware that it can be a possible clinical manifestation of melanoma of the nail apparatus. Luckily, however, nail melanoma is a much less frequent cause of brown-black nail color than other melanocytic and nonmelanocytic pigmentations. They include subungual hematoma, exogenous pigmentations, and melanonychia due to benign conditions.

Twenty-five of 100 patients seen in our Outpatient Nail Consultation are sent for management of a nail discoloration: only 1 of these 25 has a melanocytic pigmentation that needs a careful evaluation, whereas the remaining cases have a benign condition that is easily diagnosed with clinical history and patient's examination.

This article is a step-by-step diagnostic path that can help the clinician in the management of nail pigmentations so as to avoid unnecessary biopsies, but also to suspect a malignancy when present (**Fig. 1**).

BASIC REQUIREMENTS

The visit should be carried out in a well-lit area, provided with a lamp to increase illumination of selected areas. All nails should be examined, even if the patient refers that the discoloration involves one digit. Although it is not easy to convince a patient complaining of fingernail symptoms to show the toenails, they should be examined as well. The fingernails should be looked at with the hands resting on a flat surface and the digits spread, and the toenails should be looked at with the patient seated and the feet parallel and resting flat, to appreciate the morphology of the feet and the way they stand in the shoes.

Nail evaluation must include the nail plate and the periungual tissues, including the distal pulp,

Conflicts of Interest to Disclosure: None.
Division of Dermatology, Department of Experimental, Diagnostic and Specialty Medicine, University of Bologna, Via Massarenti 1, Bologna 40138, Italy
* Corresponding author.
E-mail address: biancamaria.piraccini@unibo.it

Dermatol Clin 33 (2015) 185–195
http://dx.doi.org/10.1016/j.det.2014.12.002
0733-8635/15/$ – see front matter © 2015 Elsevier Inc. All rights reserved.

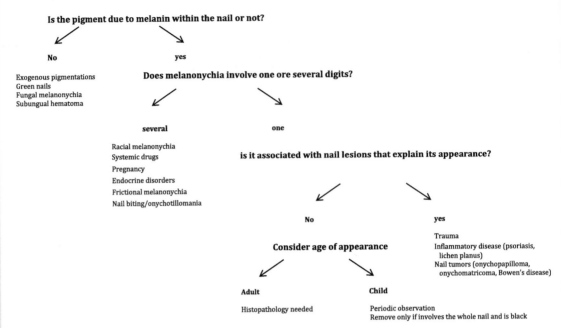

Is the pigment due to melanin within the nail or not?

No — Exogenous pigmentations / Green nails / Fungal melanonychia / Subungual hematoma

yes — Does melanonychia involve one ore several digits?

several — Racial melanonychia / Systemic drugs / Pregnancy / Endocrine disorders / Frictional melanonychia / Nail biting/onychotillomania

one — is it associated with nail lesions that explain its appearance?

No — Consider age of appearance

yes — Trauma / Inflammatory disease (psoriasis, lichen planus) / Nail tumors (onychopapilloma, onychomatricoma, Bowen's disease)

Adult — Histopathology needed

Child — Periodic observation / Remove only if involves the whole nail and is black

Fig. 1. Practical algorithm to assess nail pigmentation.

and should be done moving the digit, so as to look at it frontally, laterally, and from below.

Two instruments that every dermatologist should handle are nail clippers and a dermatoscope. Nail clippers are necessary to cut the nail plate when detached to observe what lies underneath it and to examine the nail bed epithelium. Dermoscopy (onychoscopy) should be used routinely in the evaluation of a pigmented nail, as it provides important information. Dermoscopic observation of the nail can be performed with a handheld dermoscope, which allows visualization of the entire nail at once, or with a videodermoscope, which allows magnifications up to ×200. The main technical problem with videodermoscopy comes from nail plate convexity and hardness, which makes it difficult to obtain complete apposition of the lens to the surface: a gel should be used as an interface medium.

STEP 1: ASSESSMENT OF THE NAIL PIGMENTATION: IS THE PIGMENTATION DUE TO MELANIN WITHIN THE NAIL OR NOT?

Melanic nail pigmentation is brown or black and within the nail plate, where it forms a linear longitudinal streak or whole nail discoloration, whereas other pigments vary in color and localization.

- *Exogenous pigmentations* include different types of colored substances adherent to the nail plate, which becomes partially or totally

pigmented (**Fig. 2**). In exogenous pigmentations, the proximal margin of the discoloration is proximally convex and follows the margin of the nail fold (**Fig. 3**A).[1] Gentle scraping of the discolored area with a curette reveals a normal nail plate underneath (see **Fig. 3**B). Common causes of exogenous nail pigmentation include nicotine in heavy smokers (thumb, index finger, and third fingernail) and pigmented nail lacquers.

- A frequent cause of black nail pigmentation due to a nonmelanocytic pigment is the presence of *pyocyanin* above or under the nail plate. The color appears black to the naked

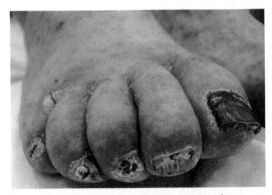

Fig. 2. Exogenous black nail pigmentation due to potassium permanganate that the patient applied daily for treating onychomycosis.

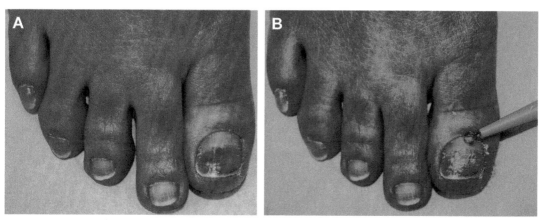

Fig. 3. Exogenous pigmentation due to pigmented nail lacquer: the proximal margin of the discoloration follows the border of the cuticle (*A*). Scraping with a curette reveals a normal nail plate under the pigmentation (*B*).

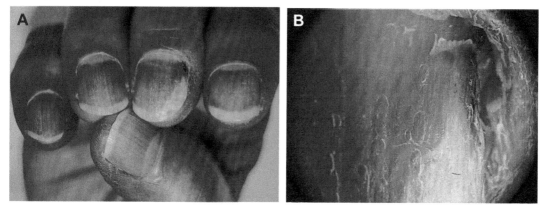

Fig. 4. Thin blackish longitudinal band of one nail (*A*). Dermoscopy shows that the color is bright green and adherent to the onycholytic lateral nail plate (*B*) of a nail with chronic paronychia with *P. aeruginosa* colonization.

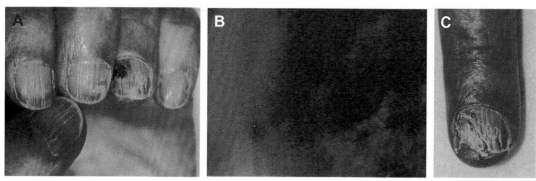

Fig. 5. Dark discoloration of one side of the fourth fingernail (*A*). Dermoscopy shows that the pigment is bright green and under the nail plate (*B*). Removal of the detached nail plate (*C*) shows a healthy nail bed and allows elimination of *Pseudomonas*.

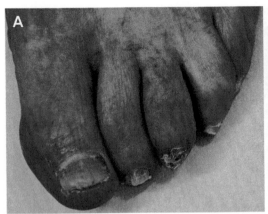
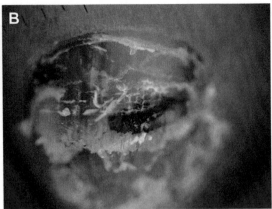

Fig. 6. Fungal melanonychia of the third toenail, which clinically shows a longitudinal band of melanonychia (*A*). Dermoscopy (*B*) shows that the pigmented streak is detached by subungual accumulation of pigmented scales due to fungal invasion. Note a red discoloration by subungual hematoma on the right side of the nail.

eye, but is clearly deep green when looked at with the dermatoscope. The condition is called "green nails" and is caused by colonization of the nail by the gram-negative bacteria *Pseudomonas aeruginosa*.[2] Green nails are a possible complication of chronic paronychia or onycholysis. In chronic paronychia, nail matrix damage causes production of an irregular and friable nail plate, which is easily colonized by *Pseudomonas*. The pigmentation is above the nail plate, usually on one side, and may resemble a band of melanonychia to the naked eye (**Fig. 4**A). Dermoscopy shows a bright green color that fades to yellow (see **Fig. 4**B). In onycholysis, *Pseudomonas* may colonize the subungual space, causing a discoloration of one side (**Fig. 5**A) or of all nail: dermoscopy shows the green color of the pigment and its localization under the nail plate (see **Fig. 5**B). Clippers become useful, allowing removal of the onycholytic nail plate and cure of green nails.

- A black band of nail pigmentation occasionally may be caused by *fungal melanonychia*,[3] a variety of onychomycosis caused by fungi that produce melanin. The fungi most commonly responsible are *Scytalidium dimidiatum* and *Trichophyton rubrum* var. *nigricans*. The affected nails, typically of the toes, show both the black pigmentation and the signs of the onychomycosis (**Figs. 6** and **7**).

- *Subungual hematoma* is by far the most frequent cause of brown-black nail pigmentation and the one that alarms both the patient and the physician. This is especially true for the so-called "chronic" hematomas, which are due to repetitive nail microtraumas, induced by shoes, that are unnoticed by the

patient. An acute event preceding the appearance of the nail pigmentation would be, on the other hand, clearly reported. The alarm is worsened because, unlike skin hematomas, subungual blood accumulations remain under the nail for a longer time, as blood is partially incorporated within the nail plate and sheds with nail growth. Subungual hematomas may be round in shape or involve the whole nail, but sometimes may have atypical features (**Figs. 8** and **9**). Dermoscopy has an important role in the differential diagnosis of hematoma by melanonychia, and several articles have described the dermoscopic findings of subungual blood accumulations.[4–7] They include homogeneous color of the pigmentation without the longitudinal lines of melanonychia, globular pattern, and peripheral fading (see **Figs.** 8B and 9B).

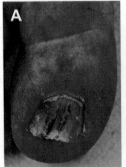
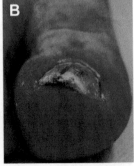

Fig. 7. Fungal melanonychia due to *Trichophyton rubrum*: the pigmented streaks have both a black and yellow color, typical of onychomycosis (*A*). Observation of the distal margin of the nail (*B*) shows subungual hyperkeratosis with pigmented scales.

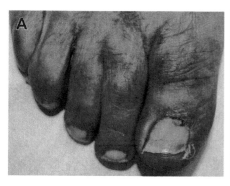
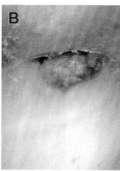

Fig. 8. (*A*) Black pigmentation of the proximal nail due to subungual hematoma. (*B*) Dermoscopy shows purple color of the pigmentation, with small blood dots, without longitudinal lines.

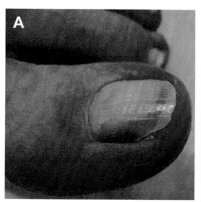
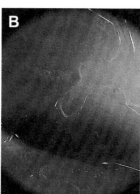

Fig. 9. (*A*) Black pigmentation of the lateral nail due to subungual hematoma. (*B*) Dermoscopy shows peripheral fading of the pigment, without longitudinal lines.

STEP 2: THE PIGMENTATION IS DUE TO MELANIN PRODUCED BY MATRIX MELANOCYTES (LONGITUDINAL MELANONYCHIA): HOW MANY NAILS ARE INVOLVED?

Although the literature contains 3 reports of patients with more than one nail involved by melanoma,[8–10] this occurrence is extremely rare and, in general, when longitudinal melanonychia (LM) involves more than one nail, it is due to benign activation of nail matrix melanocytes and should be considered not worrisome.

The most common causes of LM of several nails due to melanocyte activation are as follows[11]:

- *Racial factors*: Up to 80% of African American, 30% of Japanese, and 50% of Hispanic individuals progressively develop LM of several nails with aging.
- *Systemic factors*: These include drugs (**Fig. 10**),[12] inherited diseases such as Laugier-Hunziker syndrome,[13] pregnancy, and endocrine disorders.[14]

- *Mechanical traumas*: Trauma may induce activation of nail matrix melanocytes. The 2 common types of LM due to trauma are frictional melanonychia, which typically involves

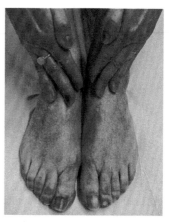

Fig. 10. LM of several nails in a patient undergoing chemotherapy with cyclophosphamide.

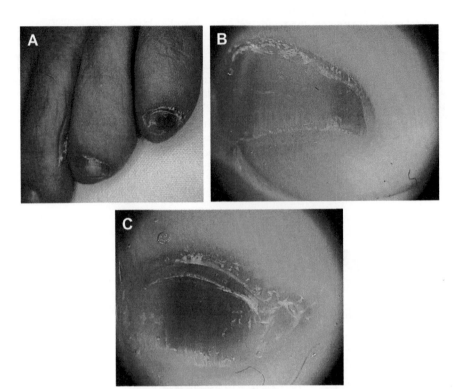

Fig. 11. Frictional melanonychia: the fourth and fifth toenails show bands of LM (*A*). Dermoscopy (*B, C*) shows the brown pigmentation, but does not allow visualization of borders and lines due to nail plate thickness.

the fourth and/or fifth toenails that undergo friction with the shoes (**Fig. 11**),[15] and LM associated with nail biting/onychotillomania. The most important clue for frictional melanonychia is its location, whereas the indicator of LM due to auto-induced nail diseases is its association with signs of mechanical damage of nail matrix, plate, and periungual tissues (**Fig. 12**).

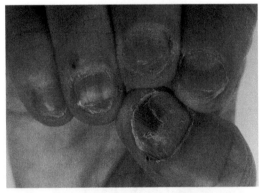

Fig. 12. LM of the first and second fingernails in a patient who used to bite the nails and periungual tissues. Note short and split nail plates, with diffuse fragility, and blood crusts of the periungual tissues.

STEP 3: LONGITUDINAL MELANONYCHIA INVOLVES ONE NAIL: IS IT ASSOCIATED WITH NAIL LESIONS THAT EXPLAIN ITS APPEARANCE?

Several types of nail diseases may be associated with nail matrix melanocyte activation with appearance of LM: they can be found with clinical history and nail examination and include inflammatory, neoplastic, and traumatic conditions (see earlier in this article for trauma).

- Among *inflammatory nail disorders*, both nail psoriasis, especially the pustular variety, and nail lichen planus[16] may induce LM due to melanocyte activation. The affected nail typically shows signs of the inflammatory disease associated with melanic pigmentation (**Figs. 13** and **14**).
- *Benign and malignant keratinocyte nail tumors* may be associated with melanonychia. LM is typically associated with Bowen disease of the nail,[17] where it is typically adjacent to the lateral area of onycholysis and warty nail bed and lateral fold (**Fig. 15**). Among benign tumors that may be associated with melanonychia, one is onychopapilloma,[18] whose diagnosis is suggested by the nodular lesion

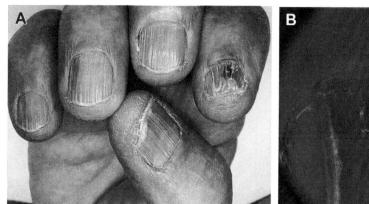
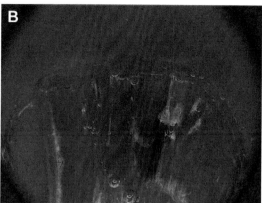

Fig. 13. LM due to melanocyte activation associated with nail lichen planus of the second fingernail (A). Dermoscopy (B) shows longitudinal fissures and distal splitting, typical of lichen planus, and an irregular band of melanic pigmentation. See the associated postinflammatory hyperpigmentation of the proximal nail fold.

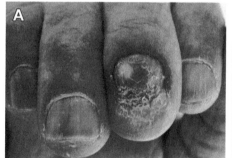
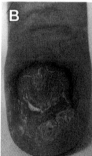
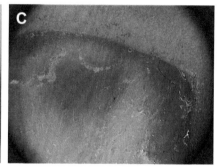

Fig. 14. Pustular psoriasis of the nails (Hallopeau acrodermatitis continua) of the third fingernail: the nail plate is absent and the nail bed shows inflammation and a pustule (A). Remission (B) after therapy was associated with the appearance of a brown-black spot. Dermoscopy (C) showed thin melanic striations in correspondence of the distal matrix. A biopsy revealed melanocyte activation.

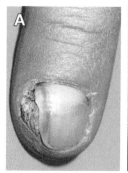
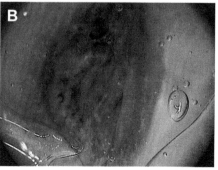

Fig. 15. LM in Bowen disease. The band involves the adherent nail plate adjacent to the lateral onycholysis. Note the typical warty aspect of the exposed nail bed and lateral nail fold (A). Dermoscopy (B) allows visualization of the pigmentation and the hyperkeratosis.

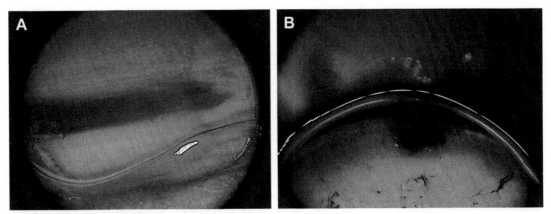

Fig. 16. Onychopapilloma presenting as longitudinal melanonychia. A careful examination reveals the crescent-shape origin of the band (*A*) in the distal nail matrix and the subungual nodule under the free margin of the nail (*B*). (*Courtesy of* Francesco Savoia, MD, PhD, Ravenna, Italy).

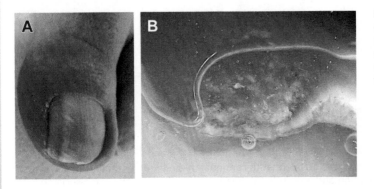

Fig. 17. (*A*) Pigmented onychomatricoma appearing as a band of LM. (*B*) Dermoscopy of the distal margin shows honeycomb holes that correspond to the tunnels within the tumor.

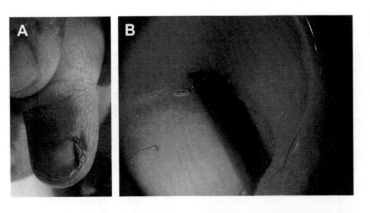

Fig. 18. Nevus of the nail matrix in an 18-month-old boy appeared at the age of 4 months (*A*). Dermoscopy shows irregular lateral border and lines that vary in width and are interrupted along their lengths (*B*).

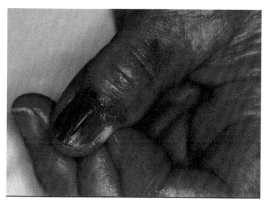

Fig. 19. Nail melanoma: large band of melanonychia, with blurred margins, associated with pigmentation of the periungual tissues (Hutchinson sign).

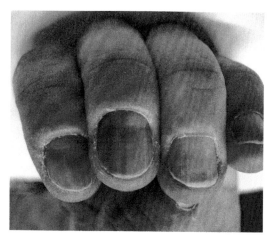

Fig. 20. Nail melanoma: LM is pale brown in color and shows regular margins.

under the distal margin at the end of the band and by the crescent-shaped origin of the band in the distal matrix (**Fig. 16**). Onychomatricoma occasionally may be pigmented (**Fig. 17A**),[19] the diagnosis being suggested by observation of the distal margin, which shows the typical honeycomb holes that correspond to the tunnels within the tumor (see **Fig. 17B**).

STEP 4: LONGITUDINAL MELANONYCHIA OF ONE NAIL, NOT ASSOCIATED WITH NAIL LESIONS THAT EXPLAIN ITS APPEARANCE: IS THE PATIENT A CHILD OR AN ADULT?

This is the most difficult task in the management of LM: dealing with a patient with a pigmented band whose origin cannot be explained by clinical history or examination. The first cutoff derives by age of the patient.

Single Band of Melanonychia in a Child

LM with onset in childhood is in most of the cases due to nail matrix nevus.[20,21] Nail melanoma is exceedingly rare, especially in white children.[22] There are no universally accepted clinical and dermoscopic criteria that can suggest the diagnosis of nail pigmentation in children, as these bands behave very differently from those of adults (**Fig. 18**). My personal management (BMP) of LM in children is to leave them untreated and to follow-up with the child periodically. Dermoscopy is not useful in childhood melanonychia. We decide to biopsy these lesions only when the band rapidly enlarges and involves the whole nail and when its color is dark-black. This management may be difficult, especially when dealing with anxious parents.

Single Band of Melanonychia in an Adult

LM appearing in adulthood, with no historical or clinical data that suggest its cause, is a challenge for the dermatologist. The ABCD rule for diagnosis of nail melanoma,[23] written in 2000, still provides valid help, even if it does not include dermoscopy. The clinical parameters that suggest necessity of a histopathological examination are in the letters A, B, and E: letter A, age (peak in

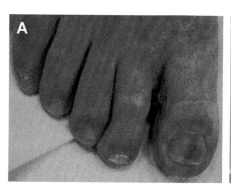

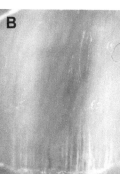

Fig. 21. LM of the great toenail (*A*): the thick nail plate makes dermoscopy impossible (*B*), as lines and borders look blurred. Histology revealed benign nail matrix activation.

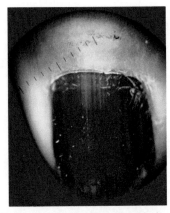

Fig. 22. Melanonychia involving the whole nail plate, with a black color: dermoscopic evaluation of borders and lines is not possible: pathology revealed a melanoma in situ. (*Courtesy of* Nilton Di Chiacchio, MD, PhD, São Paulo, Brazil.)

fifth to seventh decade); letter B, brown to black band width breadth of 3 mm or more with variegated borders; letter E, extension of pigment onto the proximal and/or lateral nail fold (Hutchinson sign). Those parameters are strongly suggestive of a nail melanoma (**Fig. 19**), but are not always present, as melanoma may produce a pale band of melanonychia with regular borders (**Fig. 20**). The role of nail dermoscopy in the evaluation of nail pigmentations was first introduced in 2007,[4,24] when dermoscopic criteria suggestive for benign and malignant nail melanocyte lesions were suggested. In particular, signs of malignancy were brown background of the band, irregular margins, and lines not parallel and not continuous. However, years of experience have led to the conclusion that nail dermoscopy is not always feasible and not always

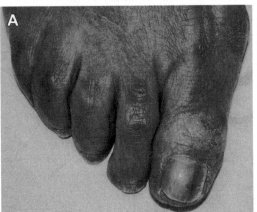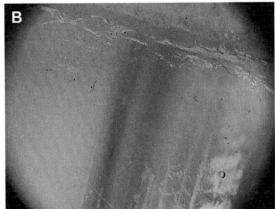

Fig. 23. LM of the great toenail in a 67-year-old woman (*A*). Dermoscopy (*B*) shows blurred borders and irregular lines on a brown background. Histopathology revealed benign melanocyte activation.

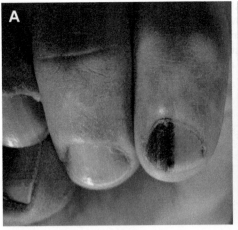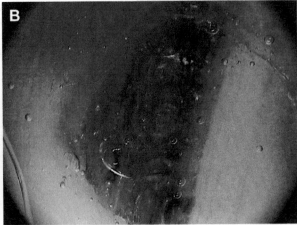

Fig. 24. Pigmented band of the fifth fingernail of a 53-year-old man appeared after a mechanical trauma 1 year earlier (*A*). Dermoscopy showed irregular lines and a brown background that is not homogeneous (*B*). Pathology revealed benign melanocyte activation.

reliable in the management of nail pigmentations.[25] Dermoscopy is in fact not performable in nails that are very thick, as the thick nail plate makes the lines and borders look blurred (**Fig. 21**), or when the nail is totally black in color (**Fig. 22**). Additionally, dermoscopic evaluation may give false results, as irregular lines may sometimes be seen in benign pigmentations (**Fig. 23**), especially after trauma (**Fig. 24**). A study on accuracy of diagnosis of melanonychia showed that only intraoperative dermoscopy gives reliable clues for diagnosis.[26] Of course, the technique, which allows observation of the nail matrix in vivo,[27] is performed during the surgical procedure for getting a nail matrix specimen for histopathology.

Histopathology represents the gold standard for the evaluation of nail pigmentations. Tangential biopsy of the nail matrix allows the removal of the whole pigmented matrix and does not induce permanent dystrophy,[28] and is therefore the best approach for evaluation of a pigmented band of a single nail appearing in adulthood without history or clinical causes that can explain its origin.

REFERENCES

1. Haneke E, Baran R. Longitudinal melanonychia. Dermatol Surg 2001;27:580–4.
2. Maes M, Richert B, de la Brassinne M. Green nail syndrome or chloronychia. Rev Med Liege 2002;57:233–5.
3. Finch J, Arenas R, Baran R. Fungal melanonychia. J Am Acad Dermatol 2012;66:830–41.
4. Braun RP, Baran R, Le Gal FA, et al. Diagnosis and management of nail pigmentations. J Am Acad Dermatol 2007;56:835–47.
5. Oztas MO. Clinical and dermoscopic progression of subungual hematomas. Int Surg 2010;95:239–41.
6. Mun JH, Kim GW, Jwa SW, et al. Dermoscopy of subungual haemorrhage: its usefulness in differential diagnosis from nail-unit melanoma. Br J Dermatol 2013;168:1224–9.
7. Sato T, Tanaka M. The reason for red streaks on dermoscopy in the distal part of a subungual hemorrhage. Dermatol Pract Concept 2014;4:83–5.
8. Leppard B, Sanderson KV, Behan F. Subungual malignant melanoma: difficulty in diagnosis. Br Med J 1974;23:310–2.
9. Rotunda AM, Graham-Hicks S, Bennett RG. Simultaneous subungual melanoma in situ of both thumbs. J Am Acad Dermatol 2008;58:S42–4.
10. Liu Y, Wang L. The rare occurrence of three subungual melanomas in one patient. J Cutan Pathol 2012;39:286–8.
11. Tosti A, Piraccini BM, de Farias DC. Dealing with melanonychia. Semin Cutan Med Surg 2009;28:49–54.
12. Piraccini BM, Iorizzo M, Starace M, et al. Drug-induced nail diseases. Dermatol Clin 2006;24:387–91.
13. Wang WM, Wang X, Duan N, et al. Laugier-Hunziker syndrome: a report of three cases and literature review. Int J Oral Sci 2012;4:226–30.
14. Schepis C, Siragusa M, Palazzo R, et al. Multiple melanonychia as a sign of pituitary adenoma. Clin Exp Dermatol 2013;38:689–90.
15. Baran R. Frictional longitudinal melanonychia: a new entity. Dermatologica 1987;174:280–4.
16. Juhlin L, Baran R. On longitudinal melanonychia after healing of lichen planus. Acta Derm Venereol 1990;70:183.
17. Ragi G, Turner MS, Klein LE, et al. Pigmented Bowen's disease and review of 420 Bowen's disease lesions. J Dermatol Surg Oncol 1988;14:765–9.
18. Miteva M, Fanti PA, Romanelli P, et al. Onychopapilloma presenting as longitudinal melanonychia. J Am Acad Dermatol 2012;66:e242–3.
19. Fayol J, Baran R, Perrin C, et al. Onychomatricoma with misleading features. Acta Derm Venereol 2000;80:370–2.
20. Tosti A, Baran R, Piraccini BM, et al. Nail matrix nevi: a clinical and histologic study of twenty two patients. J Am Acad Dermatol 1996;41:17–22.
21. Goettmann-Bonvallot S, Andre J, Belaich S. Longitudinal melanonychia in children: a clinical and histopathologic study of 40 cases. J Am Acad Dermatol 1999;41:17–22.
22. Tosti A, Piraccini BM, Cagalli A, et al. In situ melanoma of the nail unit in children: report of two cases in fair-skinned Caucasian children. Pediatr Dermatol 2012;29:79–83.
23. Levit EK, Kagen MH, Scher RK, et al. The ABC rule for clinical detection of subungual melanoma. J Am Acad Dermatol 2000;42:269–74.
24. Thomas L, Dalle S. Dermoscopy provides useful information for the management of melanonychia striata. Dermatol Ther 2007;20:3–10.
25. Di Chiacchio ND, Farias DC, Piraccini BM, et al. Consensus on melanonychia nail plate dermoscopy. An Bras Dermatol 2013;88:309–13.
26. Di Chiacchio N, Hirata SH, Enokihara MY, et al. Dermatologists' accuracy in early diagnosis of melanoma of the nail matrix. Arch Dermatol 2010;146:382–7.
27. Hirata SH, Yamada S, Enokihara MY, et al. Patterns of nail matrix and bed of longitudinal melanonychia by intraoperative dermatoscopy. J Am Acad Dermatol 2011;65:297–303.
28. Richert B, Theunis A, Norrenberg S, et al. Tangential excision of pigmented nail matrix lesions responsible for longitudinal melanonychia: evaluation of the technique on a series of 30 patients. J Am Acad Dermatol 2013;69:96–104.

Tips to Diagnose Uncommon Nail Disorders

Samantha L. Schneider, BA, MD[a,b], Antonella Tosti, MD[a,*]

KEYWORDS

- Yellow nail syndrome • Arrested nail growth • Darier disease • Lichen striatus
- Nail patella syndrome • Triangular lunula • Melanonychia • Onychopapilloma

KEY POINTS

- Diagnostic features of onychomatricoma are localized or diffuse thickening of the nail plate, yellow discoloration, and holes in the nail plate free edge, which can be better visualized at frontal view.
- Onychopapilloma presents as a monodactylous longitudinal erythronychia, leukonychia, or melanonychia; diagnosis is suggested by presence of a keratotic notch under the distal nail plate.
- A key diagnostic finding in Darier disease is alternating longitudinal erythronychia and longitudinal leukonychia, resembling a "candy-cane" pattern.
- Triangular lunula is a specific sign of nail patella syndrome. The other typical feature is nail hypoplasia, which is more severe on the thumb and radial side of the nail.
- In the yellow nail syndrome, diagnosis is suggested by arrested or reduced nail growth. The nails are thickened and overcurved and the cuticle is typically absent. The yellow color may not be evident.
- Nail lichen striatus is characterized by lichenoid nail changes limited to the medial or lateral side of the nail plate.

INTRODUCTION

Nail disorders are often difficult to diagnose and recognize because the clinical signs are common to several conditions. Furthermore, specific training on nails is not available in most residency programs. This article focuses on the identification of specific clinical clues that allow easy and fast diagnosis of 6 nail disorders that every dermatologist should be able to correctly recognize. These include 2 common nail tumors (onychomatricoma and onychopapilloma), 2 rare genetic conditions (Darier disease and nail patella syndrome), and 2 uncommon acquired disorders (the yellow nail syndrome and lichen striatus).

ONYCHOMATRICOMA

Onychomatricoma is a benign neoplasm that arises from the nail matrix.[1] It was first described by Baran and Kint in 1992, with the majority of reported cases being in Europe.[1,2] This entity typically affects middle-aged individuals; however, there has been a case reported in a 4-year-old Pakistani girl.[3] There is an equal distribution of cases between the sexes.[4]

Onychomatricoma is typically a painless and very slow growing lesion. As such, patients present months to years after developing the lesion owing to functional or esthetic concerns.[1,4,5] This lesion more commonly affects fingernails.[1]

Clues to make the correct diagnosis
1. Look for these characteristic signs (**Fig. 1**)
    A. Diffuse or localized nail thickening with increased transverse overcurvature.
    B. The thickened nail plate has a yellow discoloration (xanthonychia).
    C. Proximal or distal splinter hemorrhages.[1,3–6]

Financial Disclosure: The authors have none to disclose.
[a] Department of Dermatology and Cutaneous Surgery, Miller School of Medicine, University of Miami, Miami, 1600 Northwest 10th Avenue, FL 33136, USA; [b] Albert Einstein College of Medicine, 1300 Morris Park Avenue, Bronx, NY 10461, USA
* Corresponding author. Department of Dermatology and Cutaneous Surgery, Miller School of Medicine, University of Miami, 1600 Northwest 10th Avenue, RMSB 2023A, Locator Code R-250, Miami, FL 33136.
E-mail address: atosti@med.miami.edu

Dermatol Clin 33 (2015) 197–205
http://dx.doi.org/10.1016/j.det.2014.12.003
0733-8635/15/$ – see front matter © 2015 Elsevier Inc. All rights reserved.

derm.theclinics.com

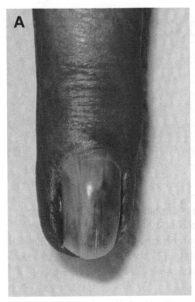 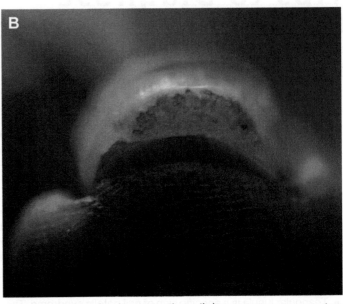

Fig. 1. (*A, B*) Onychomatricoma. (*A*) There are several clues for diagnosis. The nail demonstrates overcurvature, localized thickening of the nail plate with xanthrochromia, and distal splinter hemorrhages. The frontal view image (*B*) illustrates a key finding in onychomatricoma: the cavitations present at the distal nail plate.

    D. Presence of multiple holes in the nail plate free margin. These can be seen at frontal nail view enhanced by the aid of a dermatoscope. This is a very specific and diagnostic feature of the condition.

2. Diagnosis can be confirmed by:

    A. Dermoscopy. The nail plate shows longitudinal white lines corresponding with the channels that contain the tumor projections and splinter hemorrhages. Dermoscopic examination of the free border of the nail plate reveals multiple perforations, which is highly suggestive of onychomatricoma.[5]

    B. A nail clipping. Onychomatricoma is the only nail matrix tumor that can be diagnosed from a nail clipping because the tumor projections infiltrate the nail plate up to its distal margin.[7] The distal nail clipping can be examined for these cavitations, and anticytokeratin stains are useful to detect tumor cells at the periphery of the cavities. A periodic acid-Schiff staining on the clippings is useful to exclude a fungal infection, which can be seen in association with the tumor.[1,7]

    C. Reflectance confocal microscopy. One will see longitudinal dark areas as well as bright gray lines that form channel structures. These structures are outlined by bright circular lines with gray dot centers, which represent the nuclei of the cells.[8] The channels represent dark structures as they are filled with serum and blood, which have a low refractive index.[8]

Other imaging techniques such as radiographs reveal no bony involvement with this entity and MRI will show that onychomatricoma originates from the nail matrix with the same signal intensities as the normal epithelium.[4] Diagnosis is further confirmed intraoperatively, because it is possible to see the digitating projections within the avulsed nail plate.[4]

The pathology of the lesion can vary depending on its location as well as the plane of the section. An apical matrix/fibroepithelial tumor reveals the following characteristics: pseudocondylomatous pattern with branching papillae that have fibrovascular cores (a condyloma-like pattern). In the ventral matrix, onychomatricoma presents with a varied histology, depending on the tissue section plane. A tangential plane demonstrates a foliated pattern characterized by deep epithelial invaginations with clear clefted spaces and epithelial ridges of multilayered, basal, and prekeratogenous cells (maple leaf-like pattern). In longitudinal sections, the lesion appears as a single pedunculated fibroepithelial tumor (appearing like a "gloved finger") with pronounced epithelial papillomatosis and multiple deep and thick epithelial ridges (fibrokeratoma-like pattern).[9]

The treatment for onychomatricoma is complete surgical excision.[1,5]

ONYCHOPAPILLOMA

Onychopapilloma is a benign nail bed tumor[10,11] first reported in 1995 by Baran and Perrin.[12] It was originally described as a distal subungual keratosis with multinucleated cells but this terminology was replaced by onychopapilloma in 2000.[12–14] The etiology remains controversial.

Clue to make the correct diagnosis
1. Look for these characteristic signs (**Fig. 2**):
   A. Single band of longitudinal erythronychia,[10,11,14] which is characterized by a linear red streak affecting a single nail.[10,15] The band of longitudinal erythronychia may or may not be associated with distal splitting of the nail plate.
   B. Presence of a wedge-shaped notch under the distal nail plate in correspondence with the band.[16] This can be best appreciated at frontal nail view and enhanced with the help of a dermatoscope.

In some patients, the color of the band is not red but white (longitudinal leukonychia)[13] or brown/gray (longitudinal melanonychia); the latter is common in patients with dark phototypes.[16]

Dermoscopy shows splinter hemorrhages within the band and is useful to better visualize the keratotic mass under the distal nail plate. After avulsion of the nail plate, the onychopapilloma can be visualized as a subtle, erythematous bulge in the distal nail matrix with a longitudinal ridge in the nail bed, as well as distal nail bed hyperkeratosis.[11] Histologic changes include acanthosis and papillomatosis principally in the distal epithelium of the nail bed.[10,14]

Differential diagnoses of longitudinal erythronychia include glomus tumor, Bowen disease, verruca, Darier disease, benign vascular proliferations, lichen planus, and melanoma.[11] However, the presence of localized longitudinal erythronychia associated with a keratotic mass under the distal nail plate is diagnostic for onychopapilloma.

DARIER DISEASE

Darier disease, also known as follicular dyskeratosis or Darier–White disease, is a dermatologic condition that was first described independently in 1889 by both Jean Darier and James C. White.[17] It is caused by mutations in the *ATP2A2* gene that is inherited in an autosomal-dominant fashion; however, sporadic cases have been reported.[17,18]

The inherited genetic defect in the *ATP2A2* gene creates a dysfunctional endoplasmic reticulum (ER) Ca^{2+} ATPase (SERCA2) pump, which ultimately interferes with intracellular Ca^{2+} signaling.[17] The *ATP2A2* mutations lead to an accumulation of Ca^{2+} in the cytosol and thus a paucity of Ca^{2+} in the keratinocyte ER. This decreased Ca^{2+} concentration in the ER is hypothesized to interfere with normal protein production and trafficking, ultimately leading to acantholysis.[17] Additionally, decreased Ca^{2+} in the keratinocyte ER has been associated with apoptosis either owing to increased fragility secondary to trauma or to the accumulation of misfolded intracellular proteins.[17] There are a multitude of *ATP2A2* mutations (>120) and a clear genotype–phenotype correlation has not been determined with the exception of 2 specific subtypes of Darier disease: acrokeratosis verruciformis of Hopf and

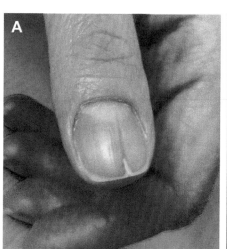
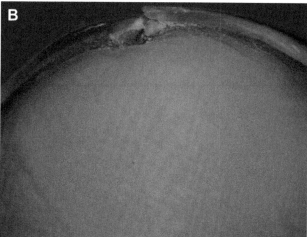

Fig. 2. (*A*) A linear red streak (or longitudinal erythronychia) with distal splitting of the nail plate. The frontal view image (*B*) reveals a wedge-shaped keratotic notch under the distal nail plate correlating with the longitudinal erythronychia. Onychopapilloma is the most likely differential diagnosis when considering a case of monodactylous longitudinal erythronychia.

the acral hemorrhagic subtype of Darier disease,[17] the specifics of which are beyond the scope of this discussion.

Darier disease typically presents in early adult life (6–20 years) with keratotic papules in a seborrheic distribution (eg, upper trunk and scalp), palmar pits, white or flesh-colored cobblestone papules on the oral mucosa, and nail dystrophy.[10,19,20] The most common complaints include pruritus and body malodor.[10] Two studies examining patients with Darier disease found that 92% to 95% of patients had nail changes.[18,19]

Clues to make the correct diagnosis
1. Nail changes can be very subtle; look for characteristic red and white longitudinal streaks. Some of these streaks are associated with distal nail plate fissuring and presence of a V-shaped notch at the nail plate free margin.
2. Over time, single or multiple streaks of longitudinal erythronychia may develop into leukonychia leading to a striped or "candy-cane" pattern.[10,11,21] This striped appearance of the nails, particularly when it ends in a V-shaped notch at the distal nail edge, is pathognomonic for Darier disease (Fig. 3).[19]

Other nondiagnostic nail signs include fragility, longitudinal ridging, painful splitting, splinter hemorrhages, and severe subungual hyperkeratosis.[10,19,21] The number of abnormal nails can range from 2 to 3 nails to all nails affected.[10,19] Rarely, patients can present with nail findings in the absence of any cutaneous symptoms.[22] Histology reveals hyperplasia of the nail bed epithelium with multinucleated giant cells.[19]

Diagnosis of Darier disease requires the association of longitudinal erythronychia and longitudinal leukonychia. One sign alone is not diagnostic

and the presence of single or multiple bands of longitudinal erythronychia alone is not diagnostic. Polydactylous longitudinal erythronychia can be idiopathic or seen in lichen planus, primary amyloidosis, graft-versus-host disease, or acantholytic epidermolysis bullosa.[11] Multiple bands of longitudinal leukonychia are seen in Hailey–Hailey disease.

Darier disease has several treatment options that primarily target the cutaneous manifestations and nail findings may not improve even with systemic therapy to address the cutaneous disease.[23]

NAIL PATELLA SYNDROME

Nail patella syndrome, also known as onycho-osteodysplasia or Fong disease, is an autosomal-dominant genodermatosis with high penetrance.[21,23–25] It was first described by Chatelain in 1820; however, it was first recognized by Pye-Smith and Little in 1883 and 1887, respectively, as a hereditary disease involving patellar aplasia/hypoplasia and absent thumbnails.[25] Nail patella syndrome includes anomalies of the nails, bones, kidneys, and eyes.[25]

Nail patella syndrome is caused by a heterozygous loss-of-function mutation in the LIM homeobox transcription factor 1-β (LMX1β) gene, which is located on chromosome 9q34.1.[23,24,26,27] The estimated prevalence of nail patella syndrome is 1 in 50,000 live births.[24,25,28] The LMX1β gene normally encodes a transcription factor that regulates the synthesis of type IV collagen during development of the glomerular basement membrane in the kidney, which is important for appropriate kidney function later in life. An additional role for this gene is the dorsal–ventral patterning of the limbs during embryogenesis, which explains the predominance of skeletal defects in nail patella syndrome.[24,25,27]

Abnormal nail findings are an important clue for early diagnosis because they are present in 98% of cases at birth[26]

Clue to make the correct diagnosis
1. Look for these characteristic signs (Fig. 4):
   A. Hypoplasia or absence of the thumbnail.[29] The hypoplasia is more marked on the lateral (radial) side of the nail plate.[23,29] About one-third of affected children will only have involvement of the thumbs and one-third will have both thumbs and index fingers affected. The number of affected digits is generally around 2 to 3.[21]
   The severity of the nail hypoplasia usually decreases from the first to the fifth fingernail. The nail findings are typically

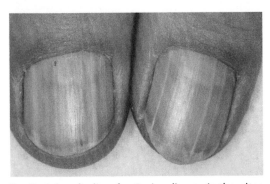

Fig. 3. A key finding for Darier disease is the alternating red and white longitudinal streaks resembling a "candy-cane" pattern, which is pathognomonic for this disease.

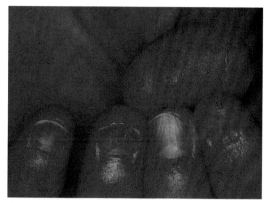

Fig. 4. Key diagnostic clues of the nail patella syndrome include hypoplastic thumbnail. The third and fourth digits show a specific diagnostic finding, the triangular lunula.

symmetric and bilateral.[26,28,30] Toenails are affected in approximately 14% of cases. When involved, toenails are much less severely affected than fingernails.[21,26]

B. A triangular lunula is pathognomonic for nail patella syndrome. The triangular lunula has its distal apex located in the midline.[25,26] This finding is present in 90% of cases.[26]

Other nonspecific nail findings include longitudinal ridging/splitting and spoon-shaped, flaky nails.[25,28] Another sign indicative of this genodermatosis is absence of skin creases on the dorsal aspect of the distal interphalangeal joint.[26,28–31]

Patients with nail patella syndrome also present with other findings, including skeletal, renal, and ocular anomalies. As the name suggests, the patella are involved as either absent or hypoplastic in 90% of cases.[26] Additionally, patients can have radial head dysplasia or arthryodysplasia of the elbow, which is present in 90% of patients.[26] The most distinctive skeletal finding is iliac crest exostoses, also known as "horns," which are present in 70% of cases.[23,24,26] Clinically, the joint abnormalities can cause pain and a decrease in function.[24] Around 30% to 50% of children also develop renal disease indicated by hematuria, proteinuria, and/or nephropathy with varying degrees of severity.[24,26] Ocular findings associated with nail patella syndrome include open-angle glaucoma, ocular hypertension, and Lester's sign, which is a flower-shaped area of pigmentation surrounding the central iris.[24,25] These seem to be present in around 10% of patients.[24,25]

The diagnosis of nail patella syndrome, in children, is best confirmed by the presence of iliac crest exostoses on pelvic radiographs.

Treatment for nail patella syndrome involves screening and prevention as well as ameliorating the symptoms of the disease. Nail patella syndrome is a genetic disorder, making genetic counseling an important recommendation for families affected by this genodermatosis, especially because its autosomal-dominant inheritance makes the risk of having an affected offspring 50%. Because the joint abnormalities may cause pain and limit physical activity, treatments include analgesia, physical therapy, and surgery in severe cases.[24] The renal complications of nail patella syndrome are the major determinants of mortality from this disease necessitating annual screening for renal disease using blood pressure measurements and urinalysis beginning at birth.[24] If a patient develops proteinuria or hypertension, they should begin treatment with an angiotensin-converting enzyme inhibitor.[24] There is a risk of ocular complications with nail patella syndrome; therefore, it is important that patients follow up regularly with an ophthalmologist to ensure appropriate screening for glaucoma and ocular hypertension. The nail findings in nail patella syndrome persist throughout life.

YELLOW NAIL SYNDROME

The yellow nail syndrome (YNS), is characterized by the diagnostic triad: yellow nails, respiratory disorder, and lymphedema. It was first described in a group of 13 patients in 1964 by Samman and White.[32] The clinical criteria of YNS includes an upper and/or lower respiratory tract illness (eg, sinusitis, bronchitis, recurrent bilateral pleural effusions, or bronchiectasis), primary lymphedema, and thickened, discolored nails.[29,33,34] Only 27% of patients have all three findings simultaneously; therefore, to make the diagnosis, the patient requires only two features either currently or in the past.[33–35] This disease commonly affects adults between the fourth and sixth decades of life[36]; however, there have been cases described both congenitally[37,38] and in childhood.[33]

The etiology of YNS has yet to be elucidated; however, factors such as genetics, immune status (including immunodeficiency and autoimmunity), and paraneoplastic disease have been suggested.[33] A study was conducted to examine the role of genetics on YNS and found that only one in eleven patients had a family history[35]; however, familial YNS has been reported.[38] The paraneoplastic effect has been controversial because there are reports both of YNS improving after treatment of the malignancy[39,40] and of patients whose YNS remained unchanged.[41] Additionally, because lymphedema is one of the three diagnostic criteria, functional or anatomic lymphatic abnormalities have been speculated to play a role.[33–36] Functional abnormalities are favored over anatomic abnormalities, because there have been cases of patients who spontaneously improved.[33–36] Furthermore, YNS has been associated with a number of systemic diseases including rheumatoid arthritis,[42–44] Guillain–Barre syndrome,[45] drugs such as bucillamine (a treatment for rheumatoid arthritis),[43,44,46,47] and certain cancers including breast,[39] lung,[48] gallbladder,[49] and lymphoma.[41,50,51]

In YNS, nail changes occur in virtually all patients and represent the presenting sign in up to 30% of cases.[33]

Clues to make the correct diagnosis
1. Listen to the patient: history of an arrest in nail growth is by itself a very important diagnostic clue. This symptom is exclusive to YNS.
   The growth rate is very slow (<0.25 mm/week) or even arrested.[23,29,33,35,52] A case report examined the slow growth rate and found that it is proportional to the increase in the nail thickness, which suggests that the total nail production in this disease actually remains unchanged.[52,53]
2. Look for these 2 characteristic clinical findings to confirm diagnosis (Fig. 5):
   A. Overcurvature of the nail. The nail has increased transverse and longitudinal curvature.
   B. Absence of the cuticle with mild paronychia.[23,29,35,52]

Despite the name, the nail plate color is not always yellow, but it can vary from very pale yellow to orange.[23,33] Colonization with Pseudomonas aeruginosa is common. The presence of mild

paronychia and green discoloration explains why YNS is commonly misdiagnosed as chronic paronychia.[23,29] Other common, although not diagnostic, signs include onycholysis and onychomadesis.[23,52] At the initial presentation, several nails may be affected; however, eventually all 20 nails become involved.[29,37,52]

The respiratory findings in YNS are varied, but can include bronchiectasis, chronic bronchitis, sinusitis, and/or pleural effusions. Up to 40% of patients have some type of respiratory complaint,[33] with the most common presenting symptom being cough and shortness of breath.[36] Around 40% of patients with respiratory conditions have bilateral pleural effusions.[36] Importantly, bronchiectasis or pneumonia can result in lower respiratory tract infections caused by Staphylococcus aureus, Haemophilus influenzae, or Moraxella catarrhalis.[36] Lymphedema, the second most common feature in YNS, occurs in around 80% of patients[33] and represents the presenting symptom in around 30% of cases. The lymphedema is typically nonpitting and involves the bilateral lower extremities symmetrically.[36]

Nail lesions of YNS can improve spontaneously and with improvement of associated respiratory conditions or lymphedema. Treatment is not effective in all cases and needs to be prolonged for months.[23] Owing the rarity of the disease, there are no data from controlled studies. The most utilized therapy has been vitamin E 1200 IU/d.[23,33] Triazole antifungals have also been successfully used owing to their property of increasing linear nail growth. Itraconazole is prescribed at the dosage of 400 mg/d for one week a month and fluconazole at the dosage of 150 mg per week. Treatment needs to be prolonged for several months.[23,33,34,36]

Maldonado and colleagues[34] in a median follow-up of 78 months, reported nail improvement or cure in 14 out of 25 patients (56%); in 9 patients, nails improved with control of their respiratory problems and in 5 patients after treatment with systemic vitamin E.

LICHEN STRIATUS

Lichen striatus was first recognized to affect the nails in 1941 by Senear and Caro.[54,55] The etiology of lichen striatus remains unknown; however, genetic, infectious, and environmental factors have been postulated to play a role.[56] Lichen striatus is a relatively uncommon disorder that affects predominantly children[57]; however, cases have been reported in adults.[56]

Clinically, lichen striatus is generally described as a linear inflammatory dermatosis.[56,57] The

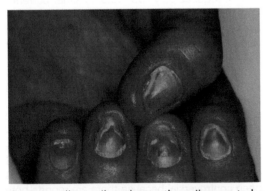

Fig. 5. In yellow nail syndrome, the nails seem to be thickened from the slowed/arrested nail growth. Other key findings include the absence of the cuticle with mild paronychia as well as overcurvature of the nail plate.

clinical diagnosis depends on the identification of cutaneous findings described as unilateral, asymptomatic, flesh colored to red-brown flat-topped papules that follow the lines of Blaschko.[57] Lichen striatus can affect the nails with or without cutaneous manifestations of the disease.[56]

Clue to make the correct diagnosis
1. Look for lichenoid nail changes limited to the medial or lateral part of the nail plate (**Fig. 6**). The affected nail plate shows longitudinal ridging and splitting.[26,56]

Skin lesions may or may not be present. The nail lesions can develop before,[54,58] after,[59] and simultaneous[58] to the cutaneous findings.

Other nondiagnostic nail findings include nail pitting, punctuate and striate leukonychia, and onycholysis.[56]

The nail findings in lichen striatus are thought to be owing to abnormal keratinization the nail matrix, which causes a localized defect in the nail plate. It has also been hypothesized that trauma to the nail leads to an autoimmune response leading to the lichen striatus eruption.[56] The nail changes are not permanent and last a mean of approximately 22.6 months.[54,58]

Skin lesions can be treated with mild topical corticosteroids.[58] Treatment is not prescribed for the nail changes specifically because they tend to regress spontaneously.[54,58]

SUMMARY

Nails can be a daunting component of the dermatologic examination, particularly when a patient presents with an uncommon nail disorder. However, examining the nails in patients can lead to critical diagnostic information. For instance, in yellow nail syndrome, nail changes could be the only presenting sign allowing the clinician to make the diagnosis. Additionally, with nail patella syndrome, the hypoplastic nail changes present at birth aid the clinician in making an early diagnosis and thus initiating screening for renal disease in childhood. We urge clinicians to use the information presented in this article as a guide for improving the recognition and diagnosis of uncommon nail disorders.

ACKNOWLEDGMENTS

The authors acknowledge Agnese Canazza for retrieving and organizing the clinical images.

REFERENCES

1. Cloetingh D, Helm KF, Ioffreda MD, et al. JAAD grand rounds quiz. Onychomatricoma. J Am Acad Dermatol 2014;70(2):395–7.
2. Durrant MN, Palla BA, Binder SW. Onychomatricoma: a case report with literature review. Foot Ankle Spec 2012;5(1):41–4.
3. Piraccini BM, Antonucci A, Rech G, et al. Onychomatricoma: first description in a child. Pediatr Dermatol 2007;24(1):46–8.
4. Gaertner EM, Gordon M, Reed T. Onychomatricoma: case report of an unusual subungual tumor with literature review. J Cutan Pathol 2009;36(Suppl 1):66–9.
5. Richert B, Lecerf P, Caucanas M, et al. Nail tumors. Clin Dermatol 2013;31(5):602–17.
6. Perrin C, Goettmann S, Baran R. Onychomatricoma: clinical and histopathologic findings in 12 cases. J Am Acad Dermatol 1998;39(4 Pt 1):560–4.
7. Miteva M, de Farias DC, Zaiac M, et al. Nail clipping diagnosis of onychomatricoma. Arch Dermatol 2011;147(9):1117–8.
8. Sanchez M, Hu S, Miteva M, et al. Onychomatricoma has channel-like structures on in vivo reflectance confocal microscopy. J Eur Acad Dermatol Venereol 2014;28(11):1560–2.
9. Perrin C. Tumors of the nail unit. A review. Part II: acquired localized longitudinal pachyonychia and masked nail tumors. Am J Dermatopathol 2013; 35(7):693–709 [quiz: 710–2].

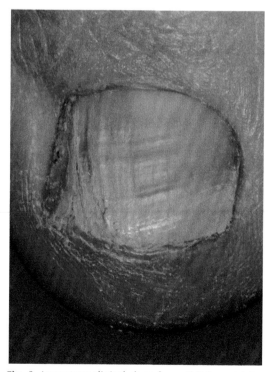

Fig. 6. Important clinical clues for nail lichen striatus include longitudinal ridging and splitting that affect a single digit localized to the medial or lateral aspect of the nail.

10. Cohen PR. Longitudinal erythronychia: individual or multiple linear red bands of the nail plate: a review of clinical features and associated conditions. Am J Clin Dermatol 2011;12(4):217–31.

11. Jellinek NJ. Longitudinal erythronychia: suggestions for evaluation and management. J Am Acad Dermatol 2011;64(1):167.e1–11.

12. Baran R, Perrin C. Localized multinucleate distal subungual keratosis. Br J Dermatol 1995;133(1): 77–82.

13. Criscione V, Telang G, Jellinek NJ. Onychopapilloma presenting as longitudinal leukonychia. J Am Acad Dermatol 2010;63(3):541–2.

14. Baran R, Perrin C. Longitudinal erythronychia with distal subungual keratosis: onychopapilloma of the nail bed and Bowen's disease. Br J Dermatol 2000;143(1):132–5.

15. de Berker DA, Perrin C, Baran R. Localized longitudinal erythronychia: diagnostic significance and physical explanation. Arch Dermatol 2004;140(10): 1253–7.

16. Miteva M, Fanti PA, Romanelli P, et al. Onychopapilloma presenting as longitudinal melanonychia. J Am Acad Dermatol 2012;66(6):e242–243.

17. Hohl D. Darier disease and Hailey-Hailey disease. In: Bolognia JL, Jorizzo JL, Schaffer JV, editors. Dermatology, vol. 1, 3rd edition. Saunders Elsevier; 2012. p. 887–97.

18. Munro CS. The phenotype of Darier's disease: penetrance and expressivity in adults and children. Br J Dermatol 1992;127(2):126–30.

19. Burge SM, Wilkinson JD. Darier-White disease: a review of the clinical features in 163 patients. J Am Acad Dermatol 1992;27(1):40–50.

20. Cooper SM, Burge SM. Darier's disease: epidemiology, pathophysiology, and management. Am J Clin Dermatol 2003;4(2):97–105.

21. Baran R. The red nail–always benign? Acta Dermosifiliogr 2009;100(Suppl 1):106–13.

22. Zaias N, Ackerman AB. The nail in Darier-White disease. Arch Dermatol 1973;107(2):193–9.

23. Antonella Tosti BMP. Nail disorders. In: Jean L, Bolognia JL, Schaffer JV, editors. Dermatology, vol. 1, 3rd edition. Saunders Elsevier; 2012. p. 1129–47.

24. Chaturvedi S, Pulimodd A, Agarwal I. Quiz page December 2013: Hypoplastic nails, bowed elbows, and nephrotic syndrome. Nail-patella syndrome (hereditary osteo-onychodysplasia, Turner-Keiser syndrome, Fong disease). Am J Kidney Dis 2013; 62(6):A25–7.

25. Bongers EM, Gubler MC, Knoers NV. Nail-patella syndrome. Overview on clinical and molecular findings. Pediatr Nephrol 2002;17(9):703–12.

26. Richert B, Andre J. Nail disorders in children: diagnosis and management. Am J Clin Dermatol 2011; 12(2):101–12.

27. Dreyer SD, Zhou G, Baldini A, et al. Mutations in LMX1B cause abnormal skeletal patterning and renal dysplasia in nail patella syndrome. Nat Genet 1998;19(1):47–50.

28. Itin PH, Eich G, Fistarol SK. Missing creases of distal finger joints as a diagnostic clue of nail-patella syndrome. Dermatology 2006;213(2):153–5.

29. Inamadar AC, Palit A. Nails: diagnostic clue to genodermatoses. Indian J Dermatol Venereol Leprol 2012;78(3):271–8.

30. Sweeney E, Fryer A, Mountford R, et al. Nail patella syndrome: a review of the phenotype aided by developmental biology. J Med Genet 2003;40(3): 153–62.

31. Dunston JA, Lin S, Park JW, et al. Phenotype severity and genetic variation at the disease locus: an investigation of nail dysplasia in the nail patella syndrome. Ann Hum Genet 2005;69(Pt 1):1–8.

32. Samman PD, White WF. The "yellow nail" syndrome. Br J Dermatol 1964;76:153–7.

33. Al Hawsawi K, Pope E. Yellow nail syndrome. Pediatr Dermatol 2010;27(6):675–6.

34. Maldonado F, Tazelaar HD, Wang CW, et al. Yellow nail syndrome: analysis of 41 consecutive patients. Chest 2008;134(2):375–81.

35. Hoque SR, Mansour S, Mortimer PS. Yellow nail syndrome: not a genetic disorder? Eleven new cases and a review of the literature. Br J Dermatol 2007;156(6):1230–4.

36. Maldonado F, Ryu JH. Yellow nail syndrome. Curr Opin Pulm Med 2009;15(4):371–5.

37. Cebeci F, Celebi M, Onsun N. Nonclassical yellow nail syndrome in six-year-old girl: a case report. Cases J 2009;2:165.

38. Nanda A, Al-Essa FH, El-Shafei WM, et al. Congenital yellow nail syndrome: a case report and its relationship to nonimmune fetal hydrops. Pediatr Dermatol 2010;27(5):533–4.

39. Iqbal M, Rossoff LJ, Marzouk KA, et al. Yellow nail syndrome: resolution of yellow nails after successful treatment of breast cancer. Chest 2000;117(5): 1516–8.

40. Guin JD, Elleman JH. Yellow nail syndrome. Possible association with malignancy. Arch Dermatol 1979; 115(6):734–5.

41. Ginarte M, Monteagudo B, Toribio J. Yellow nail syndrome and lung lymphoma. Clin Exp Dermatol 2004;29(4):432–3.

42. Mattingly PC, Bossingham DH. Yellow nail syndrome in rheumatoid arthritis: report of three cases. Ann Rheum Dis 1979;38(5):475–8.

43. Nakagomi D, Ikeda K, Kawashima H, et al. Bucillamine-induced yellow nail in Japanese patients with rheumatoid arthritis: two case reports and a review of 36 reported cases. Rheumatol Int 2013; 33(3):793–7.

44. Yamamoto T, Yokozeki H. Yellow nails under bucill-amine therapy for rheumatoid arthritis: a report of two cases. Rheumatol Int 2007;27(6):603–4.

45. Woollons A, Darley CR. Yellow nail syndrome following Guillain-Barre syndrome. Clin Exp Dermatol 1997;22(5):253–4.

46. Ishizaki C, Sueki H, Kohsokabe S, et al. Yellow nail induced by bucillamine. Int J Dermatol 1995;34(7):493–4.

47. Isozaki T, Yajima N, Sato M, et al. A case of rheumatoid arthritis with bucillamine-induced yellow nail syndrome initially manifesting as pulmonary disease. Clinical medicine insights. Clin Med Insights Case Rep 2010;3:63–8.

48. Thomas PS, Sidhu B. Yellow nail syndrome and bronchial carcinoma. Chest 1987;92(1):191.

49. Burrows NP, Jones RR. Yellow nail syndrome in association with carcinoma of the gall bladder. Clin Exp Dermatol 1991;16(6):471–3.

50. Seve P, Thieblemont C, Dumontet C, et al. Skin lesions in malignancy. Case 3. Yellow nail syndrome in non-Hodgkin's lymphoma. J Clin Oncol 2001;19(7):2100–1.

51. Stosiek N, Peters KP, Hiller D, et al. Yellow nail syndrome in a patient with mycosis fungoides. J Am Acad Dermatol 1993;28(5 Pt 1):792–4.

52. Tosti A, Iorizzo M, Piraccini BM, et al. The nail in systemic diseases. Dermatol Clin 2006;24(3):341–7.

53. Moffitt DL, de Berker DA. Yellow nail syndrome: the nail that grows half as fast grows twice as thick. Clin Exp Dermatol 2000;25(1):21–3.

54. Kavak A, Kutluay L. Nail involvement in lichen striatus. Pediatr Dermatol 2002;19(2):136–8.

55. Senear F, Caro M. Lichen striatus. Arch Dermatol 1941;43:116–33.

56. Coto-Segura P, Costa-Romero M, Gonzalvo P, et al. Lichen striatus in an adult following trauma with central nail plate involvement and its dermoscopy features. Int J Dermatol 2008;47(12):1324–5.

57. Palleschi GM, D'Erme AM, Lotti T. Lichen striatus and nail involvement: truly rare or question of time? Int J Dermatol 2012;51(6):749–50.

58. Tosti A, Peluso AM, Misciali C, et al. Nail lichen striatus: clinical features and long-term follow-up of five patients. J Am Acad Dermatol 1997;36(6 Pt 1):908–13.

59. Owens DW. Lichen striatus with onychodystrophy. Arch Dermatol 1972;105(3):457–8.

Diagnosis Using the Proximal and Lateral Nail Folds

 CrossMark

Patricia Chang, MD, PhD

KEYWORDS

- Periungual folds • Proximal nail fold dermatoses • Lateral nail fold dermatoses • Hangnails
- Acute paronychia • Chronic paronychia • Retronychia • Ingrowing nails

KEY POINTS

- The periungual folds, both proximal and lateral, are part of the nail apparatus and can present their own pathologies as well as those associated with multiple causes related to dermatologic, systemic, or infectious diseases, as well as drug reactions, tumors, trauma, and other causes.
- There are many entities inherent to the periungual folds, such as acute paronychia, chronic paronychia, retronychia, hangnails, hematomas of the proximal fold due to oximeter, onychocryptosis, hypertrophy of the lateral folds, and infections caused by *Candida albicans, Pseudomonas,* and *Staphylococcus aureus.*
- The pathology of the periungual folds can provide a wealth of data about local or systemic diseases, and the diverse manifestations can lead physicians to improve diagnosis and offer better treatments.

INTRODUCTION

The periungual folds, both proximal and lateral, are part of the nail apparatus and can present their own pathologies as well as those associated with multiple causes related to dermatologic, systemic or infectious diseases, as well as drug reactions, tumors, trauma, and causes. Currently there are few reports about these conditions.

The periungual folds, 1 proximal fold and 2 lateral folds, are important parts of the nail apparatus, having 2 functions, to protect the matrix and to provide support to the nail plate.

The proximal nail fold is an important part of the nail because of its 2 functions. It serves as a waterproof barrier that protects the nail from any injury that may occur through the cuticle,[1,2] The proximal nail fold is additionally important because of the formation of the nail plate through the dorsal matrix in the segment below its ventral portion, which influences the growth direction, making it grow in an oblique direction over the nail bed, and the microcirculation that provides useful information about some pathologic conditions.[1]

It is also called vallum unguis or nail wall,[3] and is an extension of the dorsal part of the skin of the digits from which 2 epithelial surfaces originate, the dorsal and the ventral. It has a structure similar to that of the adjacent skin without dermatoglyphics or sebaceous glands and has 3 parts: the glabrous skin, the cuticle that is the horny product of the proximal nail fold that adheres to the dorsal surface of the nail plate, and the ventral portion called eponychium.[1]

The proximal nail fold can be affected by different disorders such as congenital, systemic

Conflicts: Dr P. Chang declares that she has no conflict of interest.
Financial support: none.
Dermatology Service Social Security General Hospital - IGSS, 9ª. Street 7-55, Zone 9, Guatemala City 01009, Guatemala
E-mail address: pchang2622@gmail.com

Dermatol Clin 33 (2015) 207–241
http://dx.doi.org/10.1016/j.det.2014.12.004
0733-8635/15/$ – see front matter © 2015 Elsevier Inc. All rights reserved.

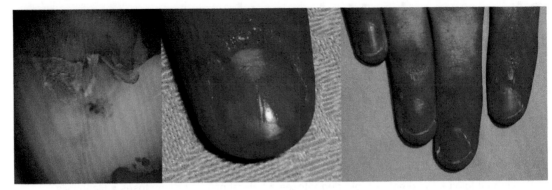

Fig. 1. Hangnails in children.

and infectious (bacteria, viruses, fungi, parasites) diseases, drug reactions, dermatoses, trauma, malignant and benign tumors, reactions to trauma and other disorders that can affect the fold in one or all of the nails and toenails.[4]

Among the alterations that can be observed at the level of the cuticle are hangnails (**Fig. 1**), which are common in children and people who bite their nails, and that can or cannot be accompanied by small erosions (**Fig. 2**), various types of

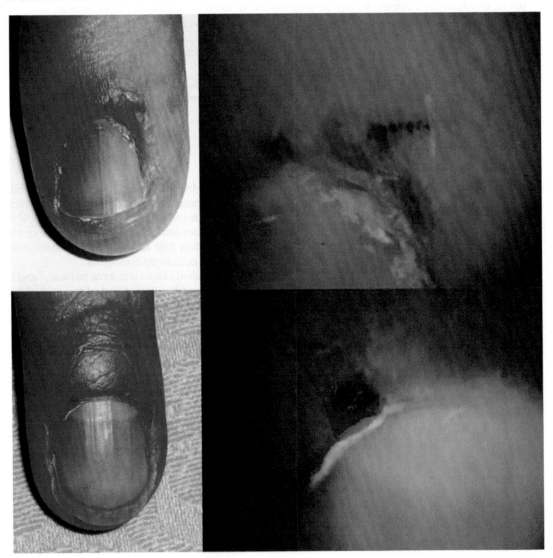

Fig. 2. Erosions secondary to avulsion of hangnails.

dyschromia such as the one with blackish discoloration that can be of racial type (**Fig. 3**), chronic renal failure (**Fig. 4**) due to drug reactions (**Fig. 5**), melanocytic nevi (**Fig. 6**), ink of pen or markers (**Fig. 7**), tattoos (**Fig. 8**), phytophotodermatitis (**Fig. 9**), trauma (**Fig. 10**), or other signs such as gentian violet coloration (**Fig. 11**).

Paronychia or perionyxis is among the most frequent diseases of the proximal nail fold. It can be acute or chronic, caused by bacteria such as *Staphylococcus* and less commonly by *Streptococcus beta-haemolyticus* and gram-negative enteric bacteria,[5] and it can also affect the lateral folds of finger and toenails.

Its acute form is characterized by erythema, edema, heat, pain, and purulent secretion; occasionally it forms a subungual abscess (**Fig. 12**).

It may follow a break of the skin caused by manicure injury (**Fig. 13**), the use of artificial nails,[6] a prick from a thorn, a torn hangnail, or onychophagia.[5] It generally affects 1 single nail. The differential diagnosis should be made with other periungual inflammations such as chronic eczema (**Fig. 14**), herpes simplex, psoriasis (**Fig. 15**), Reiter disease, and acute ischemia when the finger is cold. Acute paronychia is more common in patients with onychophagia.[5]

Chronic paronychia is not considered a primary infection. It is often associated with multiple factors, such as irritants or allergens, and seen in people who keep their hands in constant humidity and use detergents, soaps, and different chemicals. Thus it is more common in housewives; cooks; laundresses; pastry chefs; cleaning staff; women who

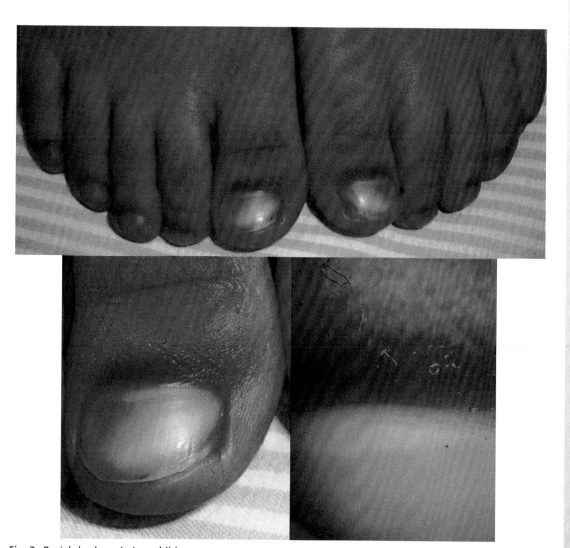

Fig. 3. Racial dyschromia in a child.

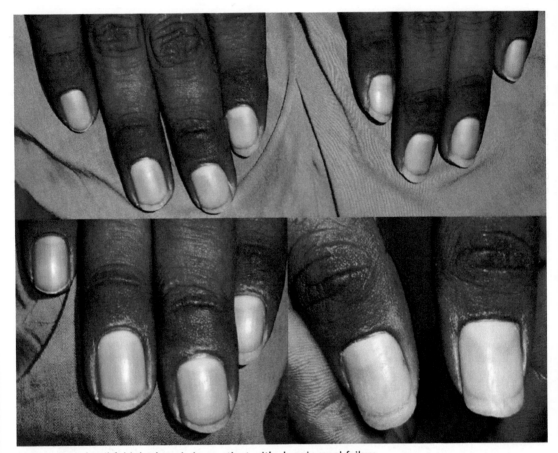

Fig. 4. Proximal nail fold dyschromia in a patient with chronic renal failure.

cook tortillas; children who suck their fingers; patients in contact with acidic substances or alkalis; barmen; fishmongers; and patients with diabetes, psoriasis, in peritoneal dialysis, or with colostomy (these last two because of the continuing washing patients do during their treatment). Some paronychias can be considered as an occupational condition and involve acute exacerbations that may be

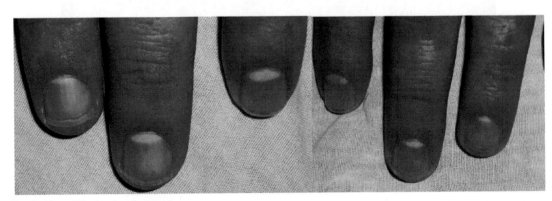

Fig. 5. Vasculitis due to sibutramina.

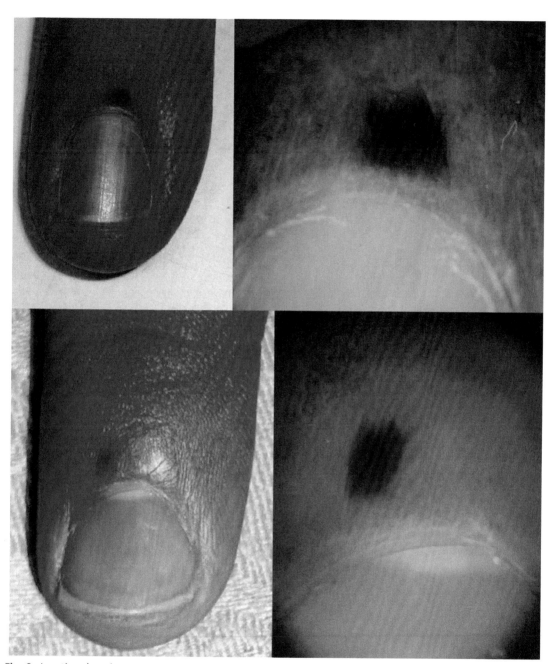

Fig. 6. Junctional nevi.

caused by infections by *Candida* or *Pseudomonas*.[5] There may be erythema, edema, and exudates in one or more folds.[6] In advanced cases, there is no cuticle, and this causes a separation from the nail plate that favors secondary infections, edema, and changes in coloration, with alterations of the nail plate, such as Beau lines, onychomadesis and cross-ridges when the alteration affects mainly the lateral folds. On the surface, the nail plate becomes friable and rough, with numerous irregular transverse ridges or waves that appear as a result of repeated acute exacerbations. In warm climates, these chronic forms might be associated with *Scytalidium* infection.

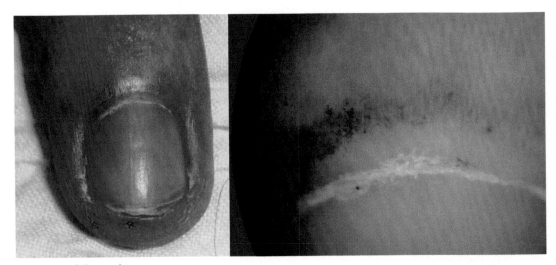

Fig. 7. Dye of the marker.

The occupation of the patient determines which digits will be the most affected. It can be the thumb, the index of the dominant hand, or the middle finger.[5,6]

The chronic variety has predominance in the nail folds of hands (Fig. 16)[7] and is multifactorial, so it can be secondary to contact, allergic, or hypersensitivity disorders; irritative; or secondary to Candida; and occupational.[8]

Other agents that cause paronychia include oral retinoids (Fig. 17), cephalexin, protease inhibitors such as lamivudine, indinavir, and cytostatics like docetaxel, 5 fluorouracil, methotrexate, cyclophosphamide, and vincristine,[6,8] and intralesional injections of bleomycin (Fig. 18).

Among dermatologic diseases, autoimmune bullous diseases like pemphigus vulgaris (Fig. 19) and bullous pemphigoid (Fig. 20) can be found

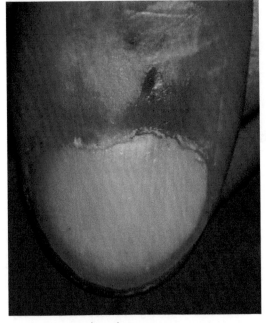

Fig. 8. Tattoo and erosions.

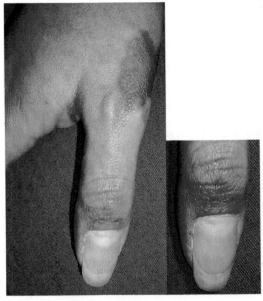

Fig. 9. Phytophotodermatitis.

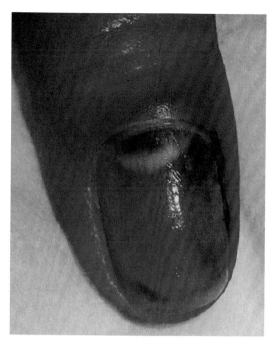

Fig. 10. Hit with a door of the car.

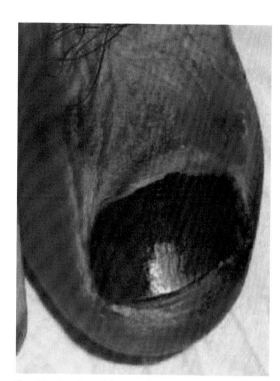

Fig. 11. Gentian violet on the proximal nail fold and nail plate.

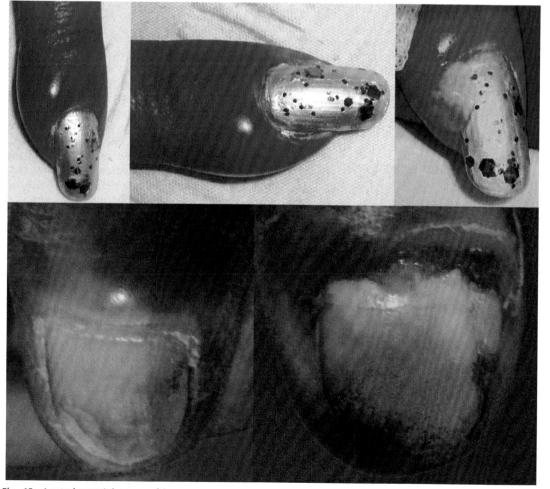

Fig. 12. Acute bacterial paronychia.

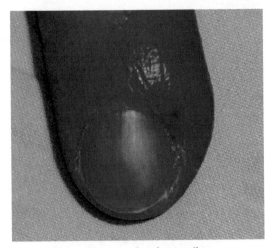

Fig. 13. Paronychia secondary hangnail torn.

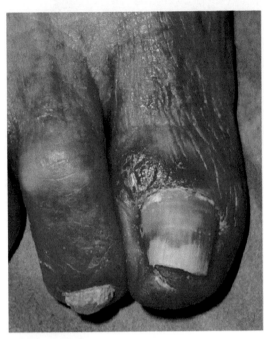

Fig. 15. Psoriasis.

that can manifest with bullae or erosions depending on the evolution of the disease. Other cutaneous diseases include psoriasis with its characteristic erythemato-squamous plaques (**Fig. 21**), atopic

Fig. 14. Chronic eczema.

dermatitis (**Fig. 22**), lichen simplex cronicus (**Fig. 23**), and granuloma annular (**Fig. 24**).

Among the nail fold alterations caused by systemic diseases are purpura by infiltration of the bone marrow, infection with HIV (**Fig. 25**), hemorrhagic dengue (**Fig. 26**), vasculitis (**Fig. 27**), gout with tophi (**Fig. 28**), and pseudoporphyria caused by chronic renal failure. Diabetic vascular and neuropathic alterations are predominant at the feet and can manifest as necrosis, ulceration, blisters, and secondary infections (**Figs. 29–31**). Arterial thrombosis (**Fig. 32**) may be seen in cryoglobulinemia and the phospholipid syndrome (**Fig. 33**).[9]

Erythema, telangiectasias, infarctions, chronic paronychia, ragged cuticles, hyperkeratosis, and necrosis can be observed in systemic lupus erythematosus. In dermatomyositis, the cuticle is more affected and can show erythema (**Fig. 34**), torn cuticles (**Fig. 35**), hyperkeratosis, thickening, vascular dilatation (**Figs. 36** and **37**), avascular zones, and capillary tortuosities. In systemic sclerosis, erythema, telangiectasias, slender fingers (**Fig. 38**), chronic paronychia, long cuticle, and thinned proximal fold can occur.[10]

Capillaroscopy is a noninvasive method allowing the examination of the periungual capillaries that may be affected by diseases that cause alterations in their form or density, such as systemic sclerosis, mixed connective tissue disease, Raynaud phenomenon, dermatomyositis, and other

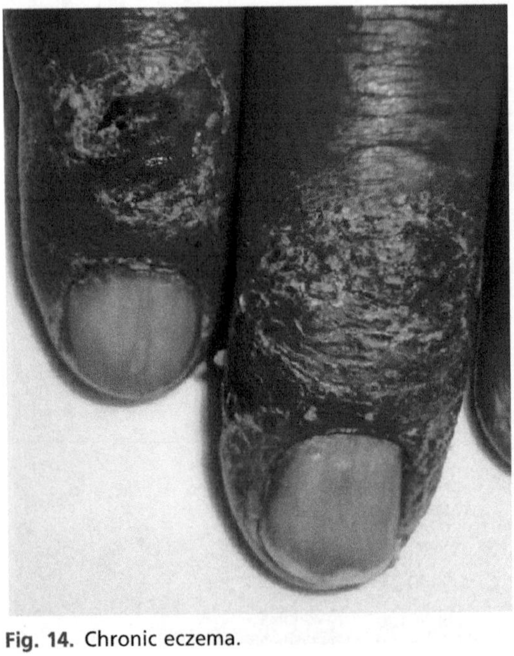

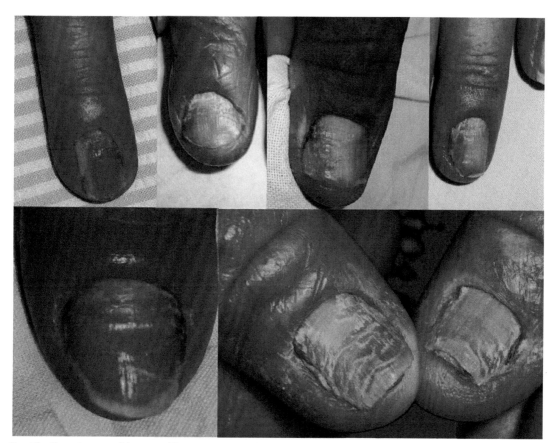

Fig. 16. Chronic paroychia caused by constant wetting.

diseases that affect microcirculation, such as diabetes mellitus and hypertension. There are numerous instruments to evaluate these lesions. The one most used by dermatologists is the dermatoscope, permitting changes in the number, morphology and architecture of the capillaries to be evaluated.

Among the morphologic alterations are tortuosity, homogenous vasodilatation, neoformation, microhemorrhage and thrombosis of the capillaries, capillary density, and loss of the architecture.[11]

Sepsis and endocarditis can be associated with bruising in the proximal and subungual folds (**Figs. 39** and **40**) or Osler or Janeway nodes, on occasion with blistering lesions, necrosis, and acrocyanosis.[12]

Drug reactions such as fixed drug eruption (**Fig. 41**), erythema multiforme minor, Stevens-Johnson syndrome (**Figs. 42** and **43**), Lyell syndrome (**Figs. 44–46**), treatment with cytostatics, and drug-induced vasculitis can affect the proximal fold with changes in color, purpuric lesions, vesicles, and blisters.[13]

Benign and malignant tumor lesions can be observed at this level. Among the benign lesions

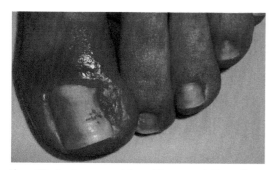

Fig. 17. Acute paroychia with granulation tissue caused by oral isotretinoin treatment.

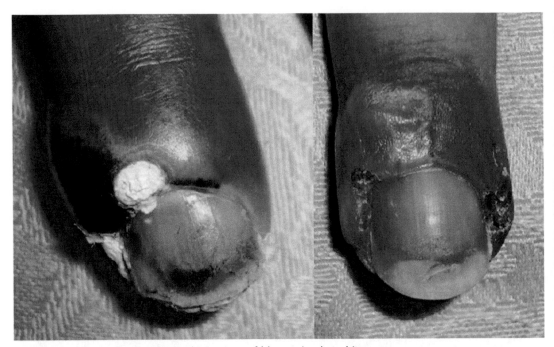

Fig. 18. Inflamation after intralesional injections of bleomycin plus white cream.

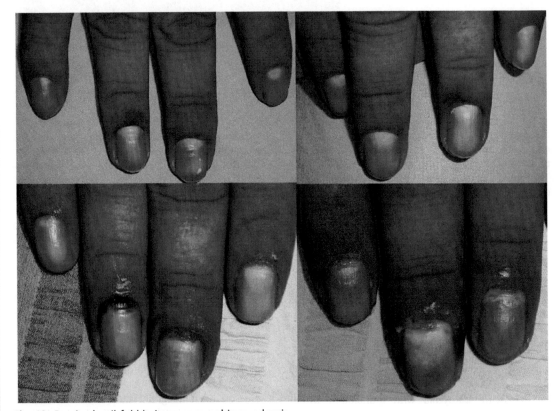

Fig. 19. Proximal nail fold lesions on pemphigus vulgaris.

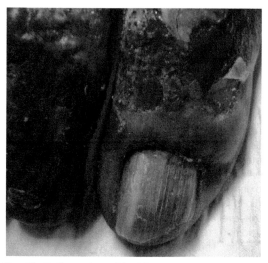

Fig. 20. Bullous phemphigoid.

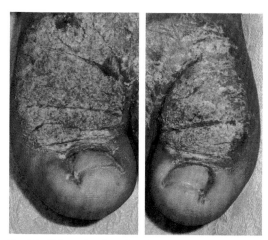

Fig. 23. Lichen simplex chronicus.

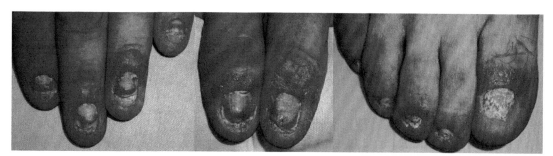

Fig. 21. Psoriasis.

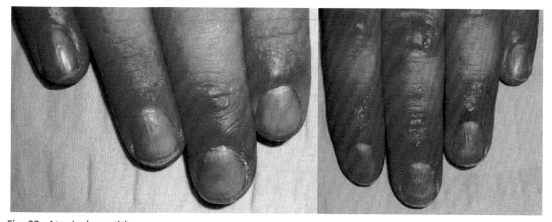

Fig. 22. Atopic dermatitis.

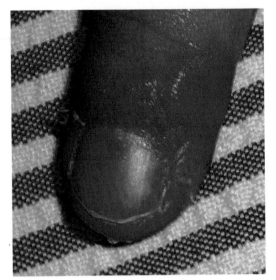

Fig. 24. Granuloma annulare in a child.

are melanocytic nevi (**Fig. 47**), blue nevu, enchondroma, and myxoid pseudocysts (**Fig. 48**), and fibroma (**Fig. 49**). Among the malignant lesions are Bowen disease squamous cell carcinoma, Kaposi sarcoma, melanoma, sarcoma, metastasis, lymphomas, and leukemic infiltration.

Among the most frequent alterations are lesions of traumatic origin that can be major and minor. Among the minor lesions are those caused by the use of the oximeter (**Figs. 50** and **51**),[14] which can manifest in adults and children, in fingers or toes, or in the back of the feet depending on the type of oximeter being used. It can affect one or several digits (**Fig. 52**) and is predominant in fingers and at the level of the right index finger.[15] Occasionally, in addition to bruising, there might be vesicular lesions. The constant traumatic pressure exerted by the oximeter at that level acts like a clip. Use of the oximeter in different fingers has been recommended, as well as to mobilize oximeter every 2 or

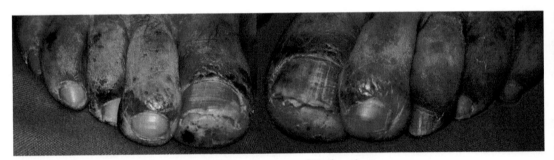

Fig. 25. Purpura in an acquired immunodeficiency syndrome (AIDS) patient.

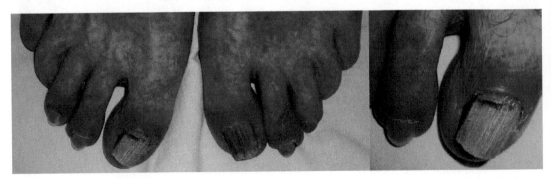

Fig. 26. Hemorrhagic dengue.

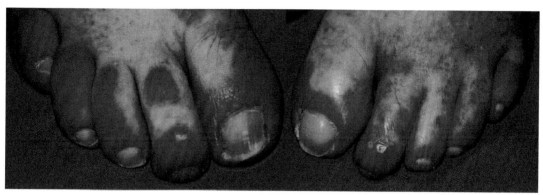

Fig. 27. Drug-induced vasculitis in a child.

3 hours to prevent this type of injury.[14] Inadequate placement of the oximeter can result in iatrogenic subungual hemorrhage and vesicular–hemorrhagic lesions at the fingertips.[16] Pen push purpura is caused by pressing on the lunula to check the depth of unconsciousness in coma patients.[9]

Microtrauma caused by hangnails (**Fig. 53**), onychophagia, manicure, blows, and use of tight shoes can cause small hematomas, blisters, and erosions at the nail folds (**Fig. 54**). Calluses are caused by tight shoes (**Fig. 55**) and overlapping toenails (**Fig. 56**).

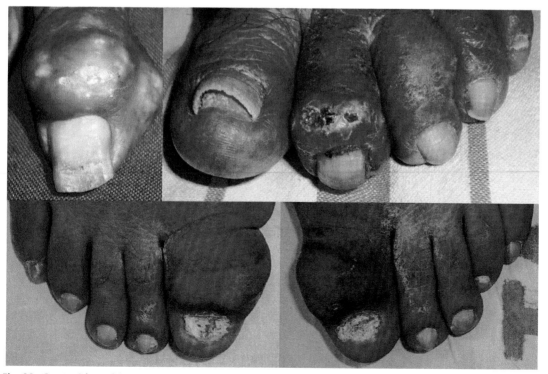

Fig. 28. Gout with tophi.

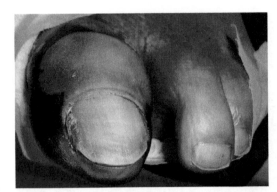

Fig. 29. Humid gangrene in diabetes mellitus.

Reactive manifestations such as acute contact dermatitis may occur with erythema, edema, vesicles, or blisters (**Fig. 57**) and chronic dermatitis with dryness, hemorrhagic scabs, crusts, and lichenification (**Figs. 58–60**).

Ingrowing nails are predominant in the lateral folds, but at the proximal level there may be erythema, edema, and color changes. Retronychia, which is simply a proximal ingrown nail, affects the toes, thumbs, and index fingers,[17] and may manifest as proximal paronychia and trauma predisposes this condition.

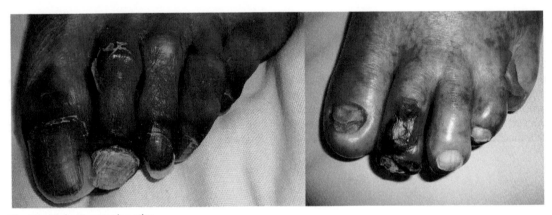

Fig. 30. Diabetic vasculopathy.

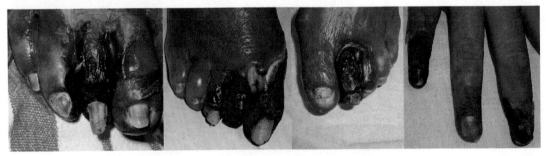

Fig. 31. Vasculophatic changes in patients with diabetes mellitus.

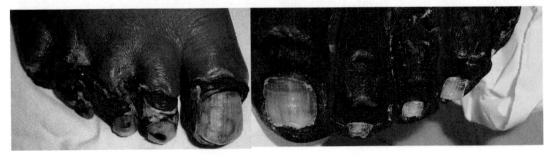

Fig. 32. Necrotic changes due to arterial obliteration.

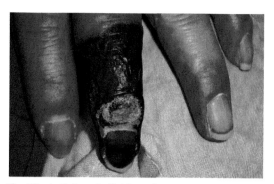

Fig. 33. Antiphospholipid syndrome.

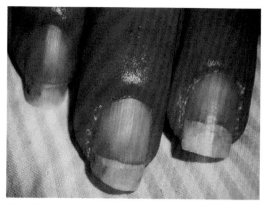

Fig. 35. Dermatomyositis ragged cuticle and dilated capillaries.

The diagnosis of retronychia is based on the clinical findings of proximal thickening of the nail plate, painful chronic paronychia, and granulation tissue below the proximal fold (**Fig. 61**).[18]

Periungual warts are the most common viral infections at this level (**Fig. 62**). They can also be affected by herpes virus and varicella zoster (**Figs. 63 and 64**); bacteria can provoke paronychia, cellulitis, and impetigo, which causes the characteristic run-around on the nail folds (**Figs. 65 and 66**), fungi, and parasites.

Dorsal pterygium, congenital as well as acquired, affects the proximal fold (**Fig. 67**). Different materials such as the presence of talc (**Fig. 68**), rubbish, dirt (**Fig. 69**), and threads (**Fig. 70**) occasionally can be on the proximal nail fold.

In a recent publication about proximal fold dermatoses, these were reported in 36.47% of affected proximal nail folds of both hands and feet. At the hands, the most frequent causes were traumatic (45.16% incidence); color changes accounted for 20.43% of cases. Dermatologic diseases accounted for 7.52% of cases, and infections, systemic diseases, and others causes

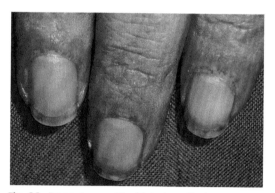

Fig. 36. Dermatomyositis dilated capillaries.

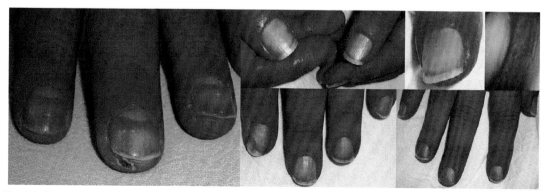

Fig. 34. Dermatomyositis erythema and edema nail folds.

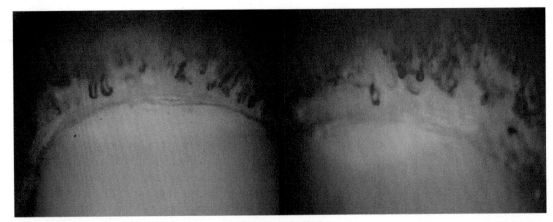

Fig. 37. Dermatomyositis dermatoscopic view of dilated capillaries.

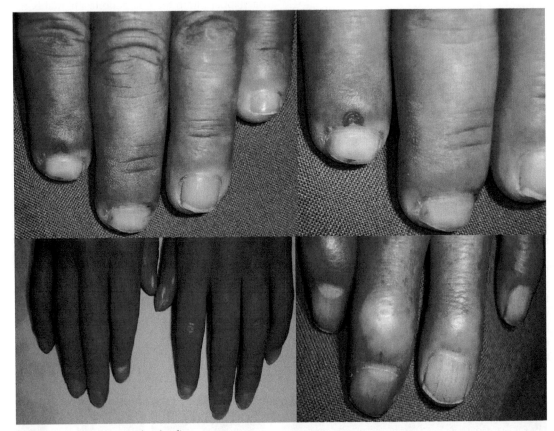

Fig. 38. Systemic sclerosis slender fingers.

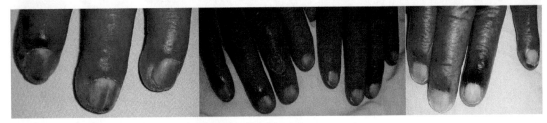

Fig. 39. Sepsis hemorrhagic lesion on proximal nail fold.

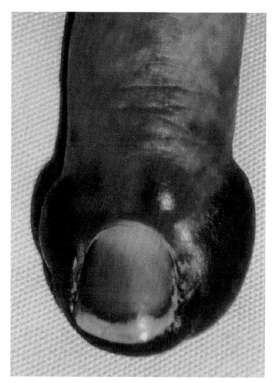

Fig. 40. Sepsis bullous lesions of the nail folds.

accounted for 9.67% of cases. At the feet, traumatic causes were also the most frequent and accounted for 15.05% of cases; dyschromias accounted for 6.45% of cases. Causes associated with dermatologic and systemic diseases, tumors, and infections accounted for 9.67% of cases.[4]

The lateral folds along with the proximal nail fold surround 75% of the nail plate,[6] and this provides support and protection. They can be affected by different causes that can also alter the rest of the nail apparatus. Among these causes are congenital, dermatologic and systemic diseases, tumors, infections, drug reactions, trauma, and other causes.[19]

There are 3 frequent causes that affect the lateral folds, which are congenital hypertrophy and acute or chronic ingrowing nails. Chronic ingrowing nails can also affect the proximal fold.

Congenital hypertrophy can manifest from birth in both folds, and may partially cover the nail plate, reaching even the anterior fold, which can preclude the progression of the nail plate.[20] Ingrown nails are favored when these are too pronounced.[21]

Ingrowing nails commonly cause conditions of the folds. It is the penetration of the nail plate on the wall side of the lateral fold that causes pain

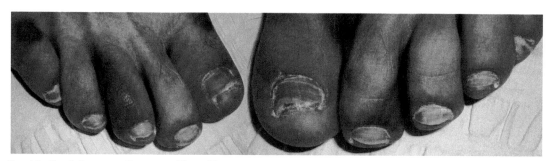

Fig. 41. Fixed drug eruption caused by sulfas.

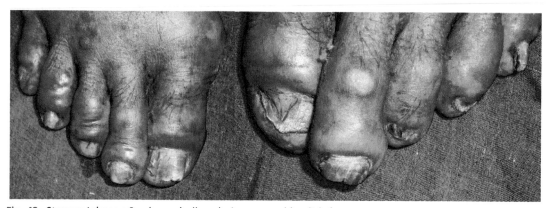

Fig. 42. Stevens Johnson Syndrome bullous lesions caused by diclofenac.

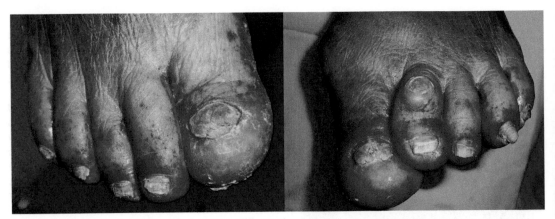

Fig. 43. Stevens Johnson Syndrome caused by allopurinol.

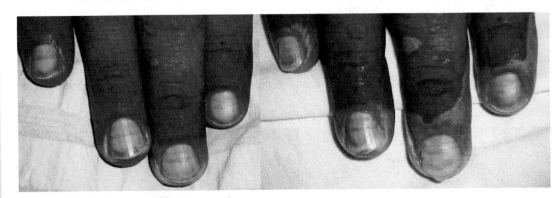

Fig. 44. Lyell syndrome caused by vancomycin.

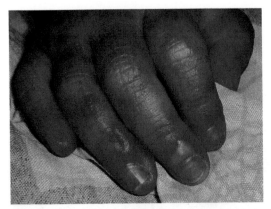

Fig. 45. Lyell syndrome bullous lesions caused by diclofenac.

and inflammation of the fold.[22] Ingrowing nails affect children and adults, one or both folds, with predominance on the big toenail. Reasons for consultation are pain and secondary infection. Their etiology is multifactorial.[23] Their triggering factors include

    Poor cutting of the nail
    Repeated trauma of the toe when walking
    Sports
    Hypertrophy of the lateral fold
    Disbalance between the nail plate and the nail
      bed
    Hyperhidrosis
    Other diseases of the nail apparatus and the sur-
      rounding tissues

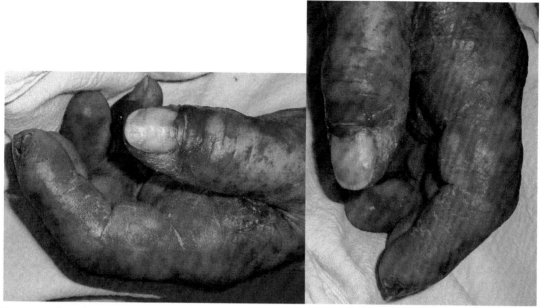

Fig. 46. Lyell syndrome caused by aceclonfenaco.

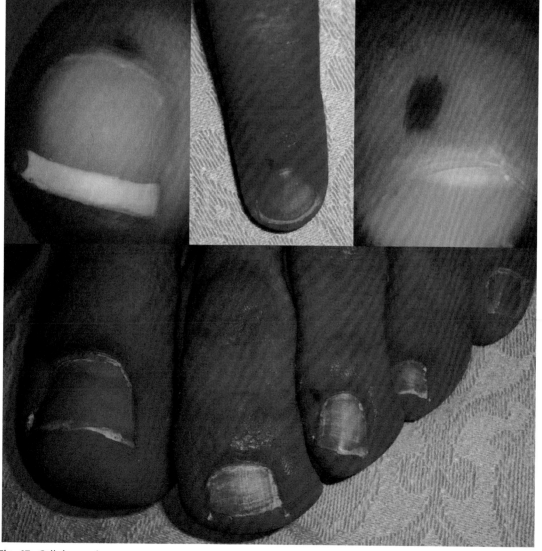

Fig. 47. Cellular nevi.

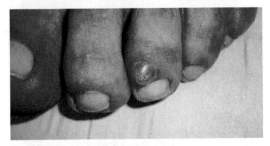

Fig. 48. Myxoid pseudocysts.

Inappropriate footwear

Structural factors that cause pressure between the first and second toes (such as abducted valgus deformity of the first toe or bunion)

Extended valgus deformity or hyperextended toe

Loss of the transverse and anteroposterior arches with deviation of the longitudinal axis of the first toe[24,25]

Ingrowing nails are classified in 3 clinical stages:

- Grade 1: edema and pain (**Fig. 71**)
- Grade: 2: plus infection with purulent secretion (**Fig. 72**)
- Grade 3: intensified signs and symptoms of grade 2 versus the previous grades, with hypertrophy of lateral folds and granulation tissue (**Fig. 73**)

Paronychia (perionixis or perioniquia) is the inflammation of the periungual folds (**Fig. 74**), as previously defined, in addition to bacterial infections that in their acute form can be secondary to infections frequently by *Staphylococcus aureus*,

Streptococcus pyogenes, Veillonella, Pseudomonas, and *Proteus vulgaris.*[7] It can also be caused by agents such as *Mycobacterium marinum, M tuberculosis,* tularemia, syphilis, *Bartonella henselae, Klebsiella pneumoniae, Elkenella corrodens, Serratia marcescens,* and *Corynebacterium.* Additional causes include viruses such as herpes simplex, Milker nodes, orf, warts, and parasites like *Tunga penetrans* and leishmania, which also can cause inflammation of the lateral fold, as well as a consequence of dermatologic and systemic diseases, drug reactions, tumors, and occupational hazards.[8]

Diverse tumor lesions, malignant and benign, can affect the lateral fold, including squamous cell carcinoma[26] and lipomas, which are extremely rare in that region.[27] Sometimes it is possible to observe implantation cysts and hyperkeratosis of the lateral fold of the fifth toe,[28] manifested as onychophosis. This may in fact be a double little toe nail.[29] Benign tumors include pyogenic granuloma (**Fig. 75**) and cellular nevi (**Fig. 76**).

Other causes are microtrauma due to nail biting or hangnail tearing (**Fig. 77**), use of the oximeter, and use of the glucometer. Dermatomyositis can affect the lateral folds, causing erythema and edema (**Fig. 78**); sepsis with hematomas; dryness (**Fig. 79**); infections with viruses (**Fig. 80**), bacteria, parasites, and fungi; and major trauma (**Figs. 81** and **82**).

Occasionally accumulation of dirt (**Fig. 83**) and threads (**Fig. 84**) can be on the lateral nail fold and scars (**Fig. 85**).

In a recent publication on lateral nail fold dermatoses in a population of 55 patients, xerosis was reported at the hand level in 7.27% of the cases; trauma, periungual warts, and dyschromias were each reported in 5.45% of cases; paronychia and hematomas caused by glucometer were reported

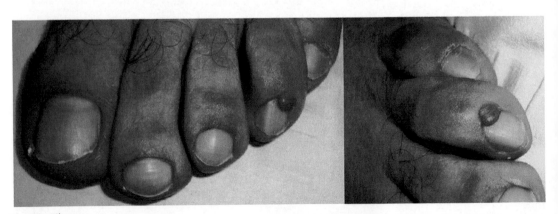

Fig. 49. Fibroma.

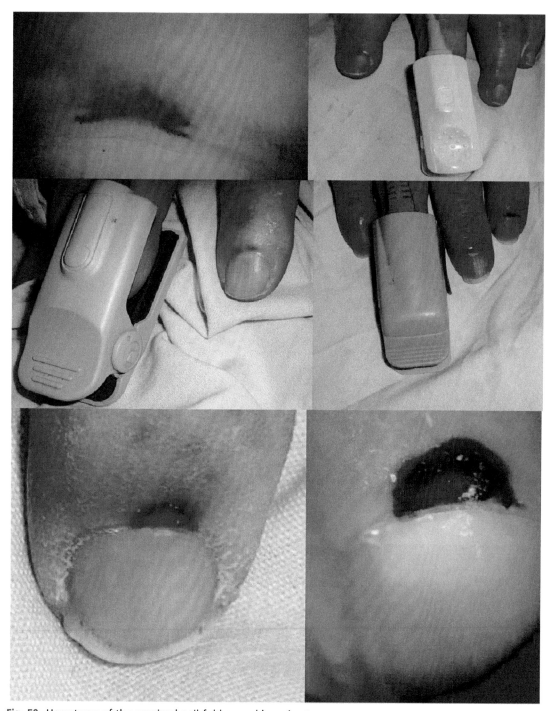

Fig. 50. Hematoma of the proximal nail fold caused by oximeter.

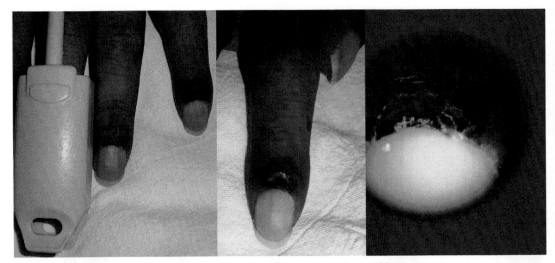

Fig. 51. Two hematomas of the proximal nail fold of index fingernail caused by oximeter.

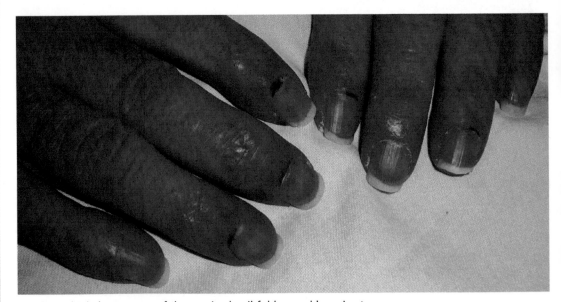

Fig. 52. Multiple hematomas of the proximal nail fold caused by oximeter.

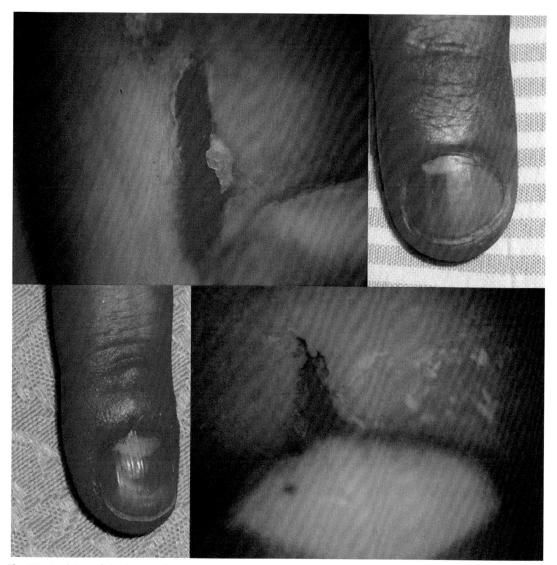

Fig. 53. Avulsion of the hangnails.

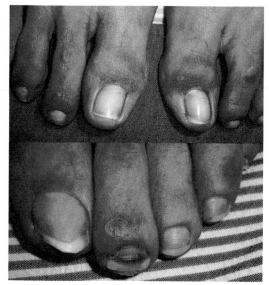

Fig. 54. Blisters and erosion caused by wearing of tight shoes.

in 3.63% of cases. At feet level, ingrowing nails were the most frequent cause and were present in 21.81% of cases; xerosis in was present in 13.36% of cases, and trauma was present in 14.54% of cases. Periungual warts and congenital hypertrophy of the fold were each present in 3.63% of cases, and dyschromia and paronychia were each present in 1.41% of cases.[30]

The diversity of the causes that can affect the periungual folds is broad, hence the importance of knowing not only those that affect them per se, but also about their association with infectious agents, systemic diseases, drug reactions, skin diseases, and tumors caused by trauma. The diagnosis of each of these entities is based on the clinical data and compulsory and complementary tests, all of which will define the diagnosis and the treatment.

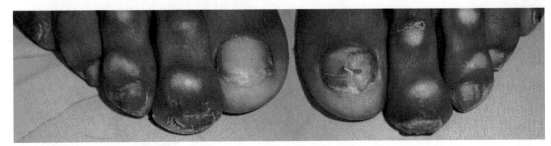

Fig. 55. Calluses caused by tight shoes.

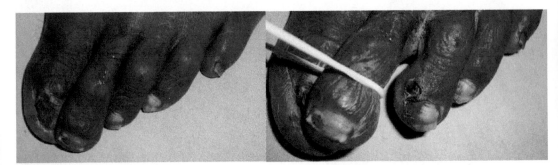

Fig. 56. Callus on proximal nail fold caused by overlapping toenails.

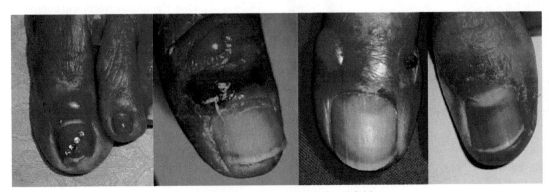

Fig. 57. Differents aspects of acute contact dermatitis on proximal nail fold.

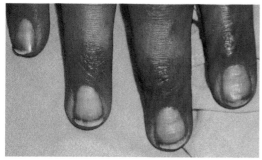

Fig. 58. Chronic contact dermatitis caused by cement.

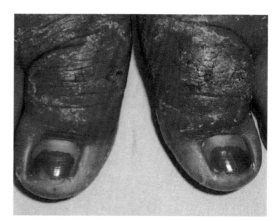

Fig. 59. Chronic contact dermatitis caused by materials of the shoes.

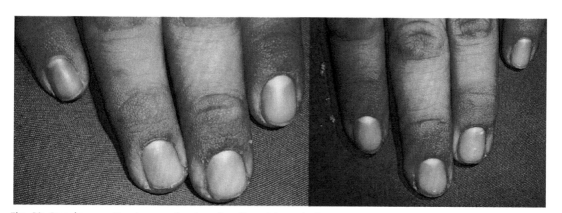

Fig. 60. Papular eruption in a worker to using thread to make bags.

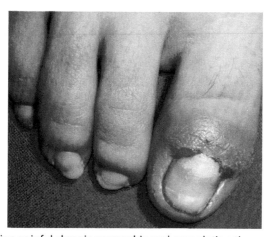

Fig. 61. Retronychia mimicking painful chronic paronychia and granulation tissue.

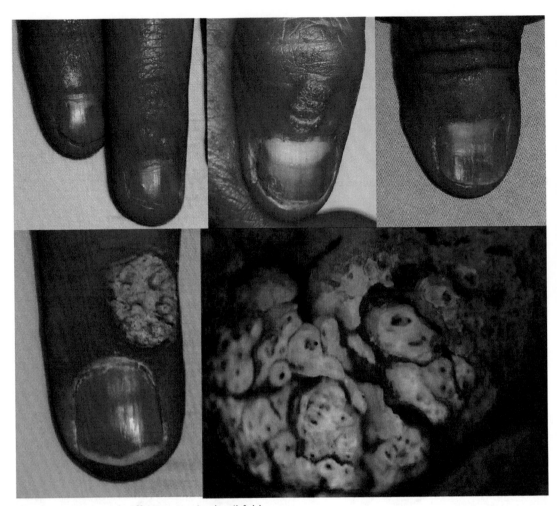

Fig. 62. Common warts affecting proximal nail fold.

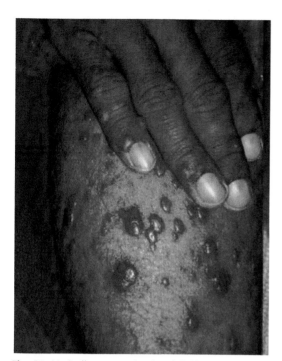

Fig. 63. Varicella on proximal nail fold.

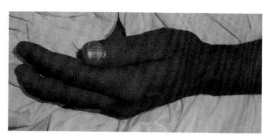

Fig. 64. Herpes zoster.

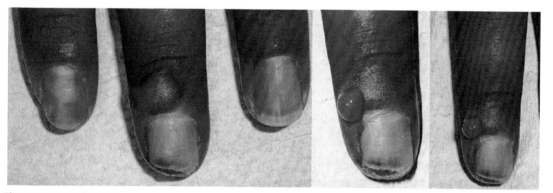

Fig. 65. Bacterial abscess.

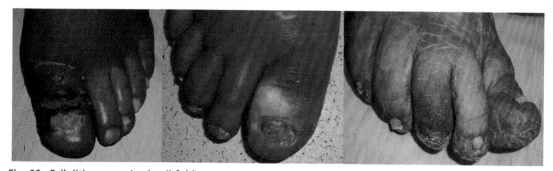

Fig. 66. Cellulitis on proximal nail fold.

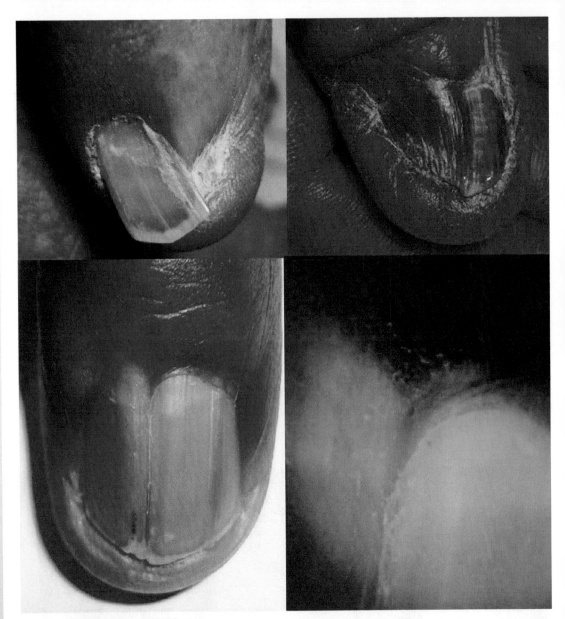

Fig. 67. Dorsal pterigion caused by trauma.

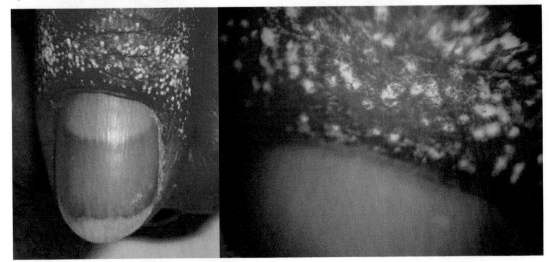

Fig. 68. Presence on talc on proximal nail fold.

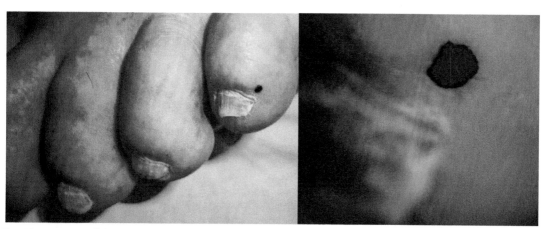

Fig. 69. Presence of dirt on proximal nail fold.

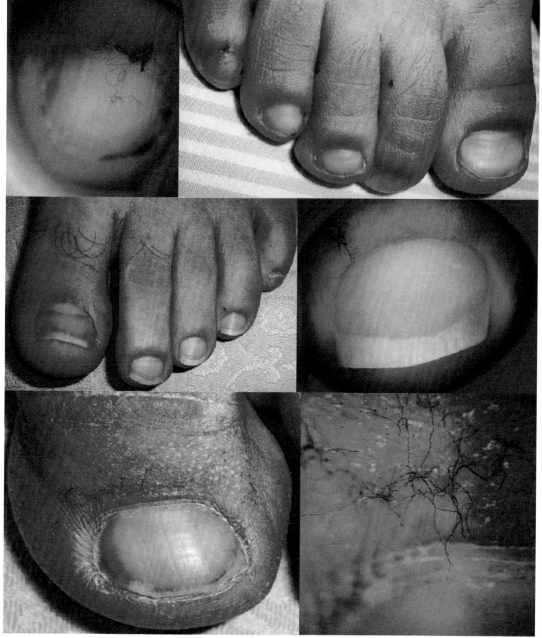

Fig. 70. Presence of threads of socks on the proximal nail fold.

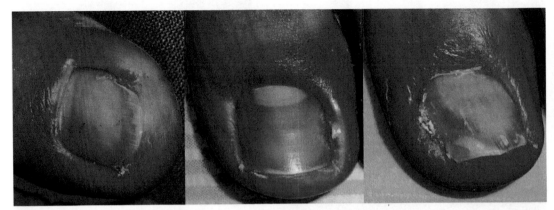

Fig. 71. Ingrowing toenail grade 1 erythema and edema.

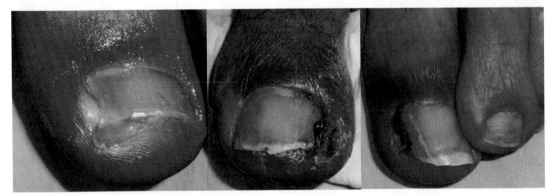

Fig. 72. Ingrowing toenail grade 2.

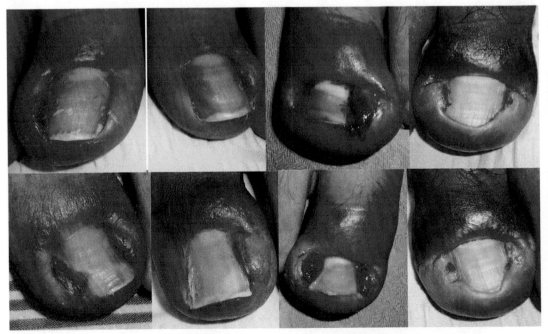

Fig. 73. Ingrowing toenail III with hypertrophy of lateral folds and granulation tissue.

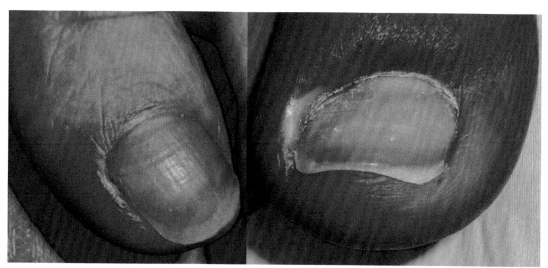

Fig. 74. Acute paronychia of the lateral nail fold.

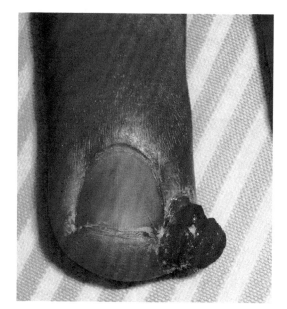

Fig. 75. Pyogenic granuloma.

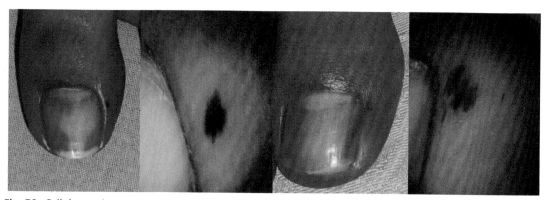

Fig. 76. Cellular nevi.

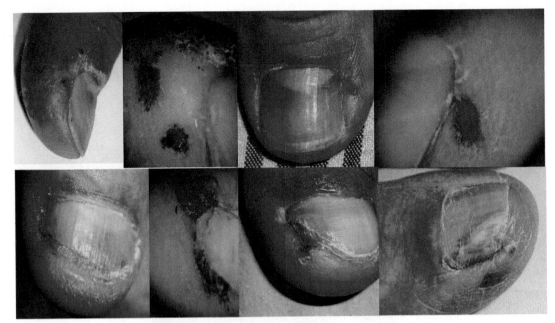

Fig. 77. Hangnail tearing and nail bitting on the lateral nail fold.

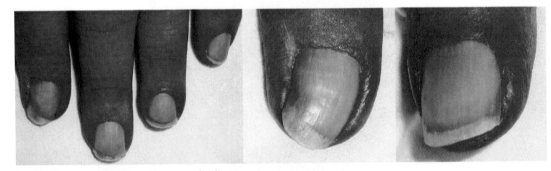

Fig. 78. Dermatomyositis erythema and edema.

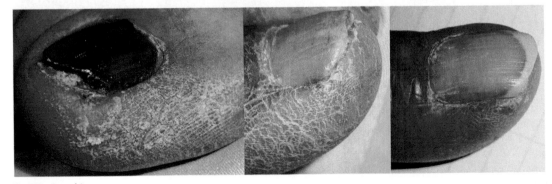

Fig. 79. Dry skin.

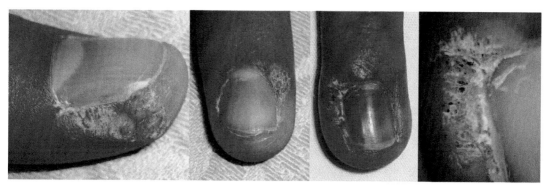

Fig. 80. Common warts.

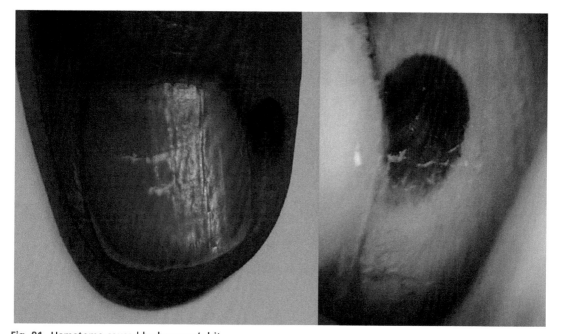

Fig. 81. Hematoma caused by hammer's hit.

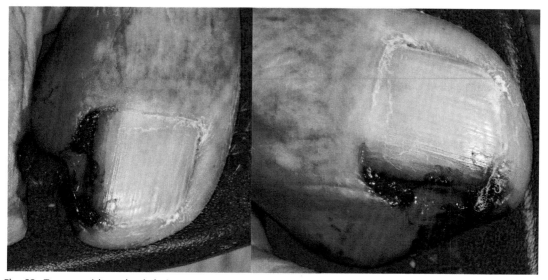

Fig. 82. Trauma with a wheel chair.

240

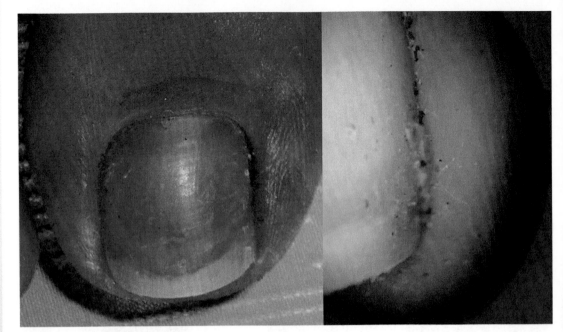

Fig. 83. Dirt on lateral nail fold.

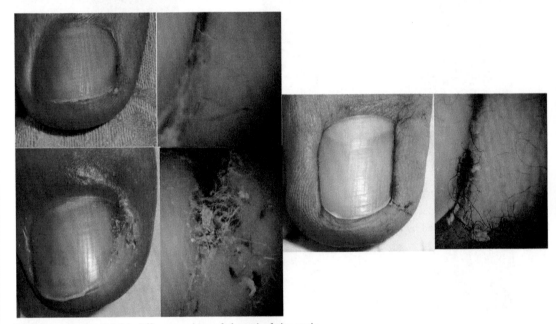

Fig. 84. Lateral nail fold: different colors of thread of the sock.

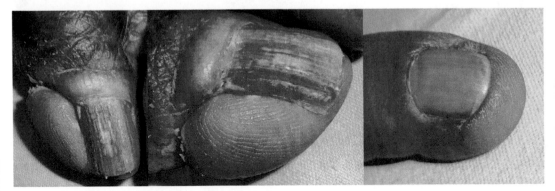

Fig. 85. Lateral nail folds scar caused by major trauma.

REFERENCES

1. Dawber RP, De Berker D, Baran R. Science of the nail apparatus. In: Baran R, Dawber RPR, editors. Diseases of the nails and their management. London: Blackwell Scientific Publications; 1994. p. 1, 15, 17, 18.
2. Tosti A, Piraccini BM, Le Unghie Peluso AM. Guida Pratica Alle Piú Comuni affezioni. Biochimsi 1996; 10:41.
3. Available at: http://www.biology-online.org/dictionary/Nail_fold. Accessed May 20, 2014.
4. Chang P, Haneke E. Dermatosis del Pliegue Proximal. Dermatología CMQ 2011;9(2):96–101.
5. Baran R, Dawber RP, Tosti A, et al. Periungual tissue disorders. In: A text atlas of nail disorders diagnosis and treatment. (United Kingdom): Martin Dunitz; 2001. p. 91, 92.
6. Dominguez Cherit J, Fonte Ávalos V, Gutiérrez Mendoza D. Uñas. (México): Masson Doyma; 2011. p. 66, 68.
7. Tosti A, Piraccini BM, Peluso AM. Le Unghie - Guida Pratica Alle Più Comuni affezioni. Bologna (Italy): Biochimci PSN S.r Editrice Delle Rose s.a.s; 1996. p. 10, 44–5.
8. Onicopatías AR. Guía práctica de Diagnóstico, Tratamiento y Manejo. (México): McGraw Hill; 2012. p. 94, 166.
9. Chang P, Haneke E, Rodas AC. Hematomas del Aparato Ungueal. Dermatología CMQ 2009;7(3): 196–201.
10. Holzberg M. The nail in systemic diseases. Chapter 7. In: Baran R, de Berker DA, Holzberg M, et al, editors. Baran & Dawbers diseases of the nails and their management. (United Kingdom): John Wiley & Sons, Ltd; 2012. p. 367–72.
11. Sabban CE. Capilaroscopia. In: Cabo H, editor. Dermatoscopia. (Argentina): Ediciones Journal S.A.; 2012. p. 441–53.
12. Chang P, Caballeros CR. Manifestaciones acrales de Sepsis. Dermatologia CMQ 2012;(2):112–4.
13. Chang P, Galvez D. Reacciones medicamentosas com afección del pliegue proximal. Dermatología CMQ 2012;(3):172–7.
14. Chang P, Haneke E. Hematoma del pliegue proximal. Reporte de tres casos. Dermatología CMQ 2008;6(3):189–91.
15. Chang P, Rodas Díaz C. Hematoma of the proximal nail fold Report of 41 cases. N Dermatol Online 2011;2(2):69–71.
16. Chang P, Haneke E, Rodas AC. Hematoma iatrógenico de la Uña. Dermatología CMQ 2009;7(2):136–8.
17. Baumgartner M, Haneke E. Retronychia: diagnosis and treatment. Dermatol Surg 2010;36:1610–4.
18. Dahdah M, Kibbi AG, Ghosn S. Retronychia: report of two cases. J Am Acad Dermatol 2008;58:1051–3.
19. Baran R, Dawber R, Haneke E, et al. A Text Atlas of nail disorders. (United Kingdom): Martin Dunitz; 2001. p. 90.
20. Rufli T, von Schultheiss A, Itin P. Congenital hypertrophy of the lateral nail folds of the hallux. Dermatology 1992;184:296–7.
21. Haneke E. Surgical Anatomy of the nail plate. In: Richert B, Di Chiachio N, Haneke E, editors. Nail surgery. London: Informa Healthcare; 2011. p. 2, 3.
22. Gloseffi ML, Giachetti A, Sánchez L, et al. Onicocriptosis. En: Pediatría: tratamiento conservador y espiculotomía. Arch Argent Pediatr 2010;108(3): 244–6.
23. Enríquez Merino J. Alvarado Delgadillo Onicocriptosis en infantes. Reporte de 9 casos. Rev Cent Dermatol Pascua 2004;13(3):168–71.
24. Langford DT, Burke C, Robertson K. Risk factors in onychocryptosis. Br J Surg 1989;76:45–8.
25. Baran R. Significance and management of congenital malalignment of the big toenail. Cutis 1996;58: 181–4.
26. Sbai MA, Balti W, Boussen M, et al. Lateral nail squamous cell carcinoma: case report. Tunis Med 2009; 87(1):86–8.
27. Baran R. Periungual lipoma at an unusual site. J Dermatol Surg Oncol 1984;10(1):32–3.
28. Richert B. Surgery of the lateral nail folds. In: Richert B, Di Chiachio N, Haneke E, editors. Nail surgery. London: Informa Healthcare; 2011. p. 90, 95.
29. Haneke E. Double nail of the little toe. Rom J Morphol Embryol 2014, in press.
30. Chang P. Dermatosis de los pliegues laterales. Dermatología CMQ 2013;11(4):243–9.

Diagnosis Using Nail Matrix

Bertrand Richert, MD, PhD*, Marie Caucanas, MD, Josette André, MD

KEYWORDS

- Nail matrix • Nail disease • Leukonychia • Nail plate dystrophy • Chromonychia

KEY POINTS

- The proximal portion of the matrix produces the upper third of the nail plate and its distal part produces the lower two-thirds.
- Insult to the proximal matrix produces nail surface irregularities: longitudinal lines, transverse lines, roughness of the nail surface, pitting, or superficial brittleness.
- Surgery on the distal matrix is at very low risk of inducing nail dystrophy, because the upper layers of the nail plate cover the defect.
- Involvement of the distal matrix presents as a longitudinal, transverse, or diffuse chromonychia (melanonychia, erythronychia, leukonychia).
- The growth rate of the plate is 3 times less on a toenail (1 mm/mo) than on a fingernail (3 mm/mo), which allows clinicians to date retrospectively an event that caused nail surface dystrophy.

The first question to be answered when facing a nail dystrophy is: where is the primary seat of the disease?[1] Clinical nail examination allows identification of the affected component of the nail apparatus. In order to fully understand how a nail matrix disease may manifest clinically, it is mandatory to know its physiologic function and anatomy.

NAIL MATRIX FUNCTION

The matrix constitutes the germinative epithelium that forms the nail plate.

GROSS NAIL MATRIX ANATOMY

The nail matrix covers the bottom of the cul-de-sac and rises on the posterior quarter (or even less) of the ventral aspect of the proximal nail fold. The matrix rests on the base of the distal bony phalanx and forms a crescent with posterior inferior concavity (Fig. 1A). Clinicians should bear

in mind that, on the great toes, both lateral ends of the crescent (also called the lateral horns of the matrix) expand much more proximally on the lateral aspect of the phalanx than on the fingers (see Fig. 1B). The lateral horns may reach to or even beyond the midline of the lateral aspect of the great toe. This anatomic feature explains why spicules are the most common complication of surgical treatment of ingrown toenail and lateral longitudinal biopsies by unskilled clinicians.

NAIL MATRIX HISTOLOGY

1. The nail matrix has a multilayered epithelium. Keratinization occurs without formation of keratohyaline granules. It gives rise to the nail plate. In the midline of the nail unit, the matrix epithelium is thick with long, oblique, distally oriented rete ridges.[2] The nail matrix epithelium is the sole site of hard keratin synthesis.[3]

Conflicts of interest: The authors have no conflicts of interest to disclose.
Dermatology Department, University Hospitals Brugmann, St Pierre and Queen Fabiola's Children Hospital, Université Libre de Bruxelles, Brussels, Belgium
* Corresponding author. Dermatology Department, CHU Brugmann, Place Van Gehuchten, 4, Brussels 1020, Belgium.
E-mail address: bertrand.richert@chu-brugmann.be

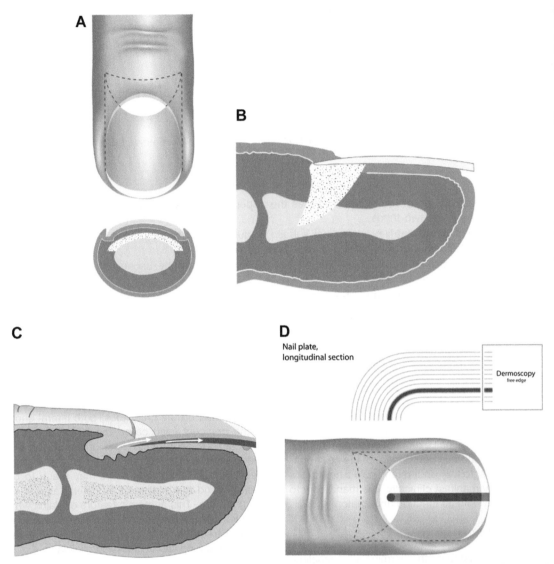

Fig. 1. (*A*) Position of the matrix on a digit. (*B*) Position of the matrix on a great toenail. Note how the lateral horns of the matrix expand laterally. (*C*) Production of the nail plate by the 2 matrix compartments. (*D*) Correlation between the position of a pigmented band within the matrix and its location on the free edge. (*Courtesy of Florence Richert, Bordeaux Mérignac, France.*)

2. Nail matrix melanocytes are 6 times less numerous in the matrix ($200/mm^2$) than in the skin epidermis ($1200/mm^2$). Their numbers are similar in the proximal and the distal matrix, but they differ in their usual quiescence: in the proximal matrix, most matrix melanocytes are dormant and do not produce any pigment whereas in the distal matrix 50% are dormant and 50% are activable.[4] When activated, they synthesize melanin, which is transferred to the surrounding keratinocytes. Distal migration of melanin-containing keratinocytes gives rise to a pigmented nail plate. For this reason, most longitudinal melanonychias arise in the distal matrix,[4] which is fortunate if they have to be surgically removed (discussed later).

FORMATION OF THE NAIL PLATE

1. The matrix creates all or most of the nail plate.[5] The proximal portion of the matrix produces the upper third of the nail plate and its distal part produces the lower two-thirds (see **Fig. 1**C).[6] This feature is important in nail surgery: removing a part of the distal matrix (eg, with a punch) does not lead to nail dystrophy because the defect will be covered by the upper part of the plate synthesized by the proximal matrix (see **Fig. 1**D).

2. The thickness of the nail plate is proportional to the length of the matrix (thumbnails and great toenails are thicker).
3. The shape of the lunula determines the contour of the free edge.[6]

GROWTH OF THE NAIL PLATE

The average fingernail growth rate (3.47 mm/mo) is more than twice as fast as that of the toenail (1.62 mm/mo).[7–9] This rate has increased over the last 30 years thanks to the improvement in quality of life, health conditions, and diet.[7] This growth rate allows clinicians to date an event that left a nail surface dystrophy (eg, Beau line, hematoma) by measuring the distance between the cuticle and the dystrophy.

CLINICAL SIGNS OF NAIL MATRIX INSULTS

The resultant nail signs depend on the intensity (mild, moderate, or severe), the duration (transient or prolonged), and the extent (focal, widespread) of the insult.[1]

Because the proximal matrix synthesizes the upper part of the nail plate, an insult to the proximal matrix produces nail surface irregularities: longitudinal lines, transverse lines, roughness of the nail surface, pitting, or superficial brittleness.

When the distal matrix is affected, the condition may present as a longitudinal, transverse, or diffuse chromonychia (melanonychia, erythronychia, leukonychia).

CLINICAL SIGNS OF PROXIMAL MATRIX INVOLVEMENT
Longitudinal Lines May Appear as Projecting Ridges or Indented Grooves

Longitudinal ridging
Multiple shallow and delicate longitudinal ridging is physiologic. This relief becomes more prominent with aging (**Fig. 2**). The ridges may be focally interrupted, giving rise to a beaded appearance. In contrast with what is noted in young adults, there is a discrepancy and an irregularity in the turnover of the matrix cells. These variations are probably responsible for the exaggeration of the longitudinal ridges observed on senile nails.[10] Ridges may also be observed in some pathologic states, such as rheumatoid arthritis, peripheral vascular disorders, and Darier disease.[6]

Sometimes both thumbs have a wide median longitudinal ridge that has the shape of a circumflex accent in cross section. This condition may be inherited or, if acquired, is posttraumatic.[6]

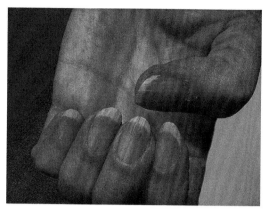

Fig. 2. Accentuation of the longitudinal ridging with age.

Longitudinal grooves
These depressions may run on a part or on the whole nail length. They can be single, multiple, on 1 or several nails, and are associated with a pathologic state in almost all instances. They arise from a focal prolonged moderate insult to the proximal matrix.[1] Depending on the depth, length, and width of the depression, clinicians talk about fissures (narrow and superficial), cracks (short, deep and narrow), splits (long, deep, and narrow), grooves (wide, long and deep), or gutters (larger grooves).

Onychorrhexis defines multiple superficial fissures that give the appearance of the nail having been scratched with coarse sandpaper or with an awl. Some splits may be associated. These fissures are the most common presentation of lichen planus (**Fig. 3**).

The median canaliform dystrophy of Heller is characterized by a midline inverted fir tree–like crack emerging from under the cuticle and extending up to two-thirds of the proximal nail plate (**Fig. 4**). It rarely reaches the free edge. This

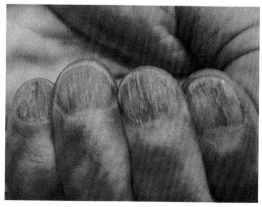

Fig. 3. Onychorrhexis.

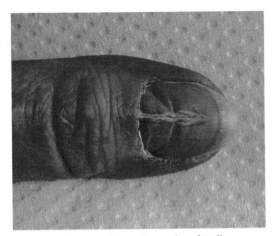

Fig. 4. Median canaliform dystrophy of Heller.

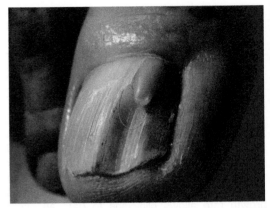

Fig. 6. Fibrokeratoma emerging under the proximal nail fold and resting in a smooth gutter.

dystrophy electively affects the thumbnails. Its cause remains unclear and it is probably a self-inflicted repeated pressure on the proximal region[11] of the nail, as indicated by the enlarged lunula and its disappearance with protection of the proximal nail. Two cases have been attributed to isotretinoin, both improving on withdrawal of the drug.[12,13]

A single smooth and harmonious longitudinal gutter results from prolonged focal pressure on the underlying matrix by a tumor located on or under the proximal nail fold. These tumors are mainly benign: myxoid pseudocyst (Fig. 5), fibrokeratoma (Fig. 6), implantation cyst, wart, and giant-cell tumor of the tendon sheath. Myxoid pseudocysts usually imprint a smooth wide gutter on the plate. However, some may vary in size: inflammation or drainage temporarily lessens their pressure on the matrix before they swell again. This process results in a typical irregular groove of varying depths (Fig. 7). No other tumor varies

in size. The main causes of longitudinal lines are listed in **Table 1**.

Transverse Lines Are Always Grooves

Transverse grooves originating from the matrix always parallel the distal edge of the lunula. Transverse grooves following the curve of the proximal nail fold have an exogenous origin (eg, manicuring) (**Fig. 8**). The French physician Joseph Honoré Simon Beau first described this nail dystrophy in 1846 after typhoid fever and other acute systemic diseases. Beau was a cardiologist, but the medical community remembers him for noticing this condition. The groove results from a transient decrease of the matrix mitotic activity, resulting in a focal thinning of the nail plate. The groove is more pronounced in the middle part of the nail. Beau lines emerge from under the cuticle 4 to 8 weeks after the matrix insult[14]; they grow out distally with the nail growth. Because the nail plate grows at a

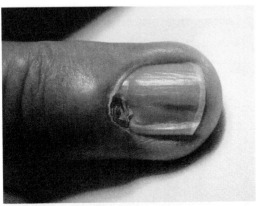

Fig. 5. Myxoid pseudocyst. Note the smooth groove facing the lesion.

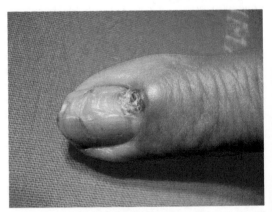

Fig. 7. Irregular longitudinal gutter from a myxoid pseudocyst varying in size over time.

Table 1
Principal causes of longitudinal lines

Single median fissure	Trauma Median canaliform dystrophy of Heller
Gutter	Tumor of the proximal nail fold
Onychorrhexis	Lichen planus Rheumatoid arthritis Raynaud disease
Multiple longitudinal ridges	Physiologic Old age Rheumatoid arthritis

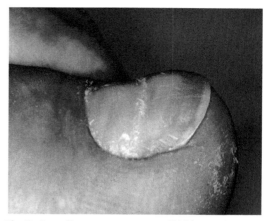

Fig. 9. Beau line on a great toenail (side view), resulting from too-tight ski boots during winter holidays, 6 months before.

speed of 0.10 mm/d, it is easy retrospectively to estimate the timing of the causal event by measuring the distance between the groove and the proximal nail fold. One single transverse groove on 1 nail is secondary to a local phenomenon (eg, trauma) (**Fig. 9**). The existence of 1 groove on several nails, at the same level, reflects a systemic event. Several Beau lines on all nails suggest a repeated insult to the matrix (eg, chemotherapy) (**Fig. 10**).[15] Neonates may show Beau lines at 8 to 9 weeks of age, reflecting the transition from intrauterine to extrauterine life.[16] The main causes for Beau lines are listed in **Table 2**.

Onychomadesis refers to a proximal detachment of the plate followed by nail shedding. It appears after an insult to the proximal matrix that lasts for more than 1 or 2 weeks or after a complete arrest of the matrix activity. A new nail is formed and slides under the former nail, which is lifted up and pushed away. Onychomadesis has gain popularity lasting recent years from

epidemic outbreaks of hand-foot-and-mouth syndrome associated with this nail dystrophy (**Fig. 11**).[17–23]

Multiple parallel transverse grooves, especially on the thumbnails, spreading from the cuticle up to the free edge, located in the middle of the plate and giving rise to a characteristic washboard aspect, indicate a self-induced dystrophy. This condition is called habit tic and the dystrophy comes from the repeated pushing back of the cuticle from the thumb with the nail of the index or middle finger of the same hand or the contralateral thumbnail.[24,25] This habit leads to transient repeated widespread insult to the matrix, resulting each time in a moderately deep transverse groove. If the habit exerts a sufficient and constant strong pressure on the proximal area, it also leads to a wide longitudinal groove where the transverse grooves rest (**Figs. 12** and **13**). Pressure induces an enlargement of the lunula (macrolunula), which is an excellent diagnostic clue. Cuticles may be

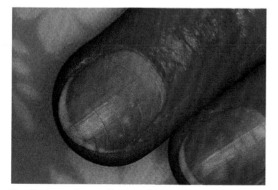

Fig. 8. Curved scratches on the nail plate paralleling the curve of the proximal nail fold: manicuring induced. Each scratch correspond with 1 manicure, it can easy be calculated that there is about 4 weeks between each manicure.

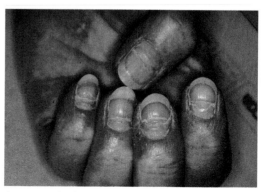

Fig. 10. Multiple Beau lines at the same level in a patient under cyclic chemotherapies.

Table 2
Principal causes of transverse grooves (Beau lines)

Polydactylous single groove	Birth Infectious disease Feverish disease
Monodactylous single groove	Trauma Surgery Acute paronychia Carpal tunnel syndrome
Monodactylous multiple grooves	Habit tic deformity (thumbs almost exclusively) Chronic paronychia
Polydactylous multiple grooves	Regular cosmetic traumatism Retinoids Eczema Successive chemotherapies

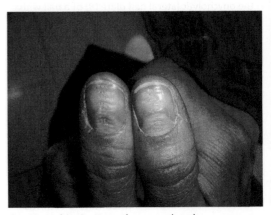

Fig. 12. Habit tic. Note the macrolunula.

partially or totally absent and a subacute paronychia may be associated. A habit tic was recently associated with guitar playing,[26] and in one case it was responsible for an added elkonyxis.[27]

Pitting

Pitting describes the presence of small depressions on the nail plate surface. Pits are foci of abnormal keratinization of the proximal nail matrix, which results in clusters of parakeratotic cells in the dorsal nail plate. These clusters are easily detached, leaving the pits. These depressions are variable in size, shape, width, and depth depending on the duration and extent of matrix involvement. They may be distributed randomly, along longitudinal lines, or in a rippled pattern (**Fig. 14**).[1,6] Pits are unusual on toenails.

Pits are highly suggestive but not pathognomonic of psoriasis. Psoriatic nail pits are usually deep and scattered randomly, but occasionally they occur in a longitudinal ridge or gridlike pattern. It has been stated that greater than 20 fingernail pits suggests psoriasis.[6] In nail psoriasis, pitting is the most common clinical feature: it occurs in two-thirds of adults[28] and children.[29]

In alopecia areata, pitting is the most frequent anomaly, especially in children; one-third of young patients with alopecia areata, totalis, or universalis had nail pitting in one study.[30] The pits are small, shallow, and more diffuse compared with psoriatic pits (**Fig. 15**). The pattern is often regular or rippled geometric rows, or longitudinal lines.[6] The significance is unknown, and whether this is a poor prognostic indicator for regrowth remains controversial. Pits may precede or follow the onset of alopecia, and may persist after regrowth.

The other common causes include eczema and occupational trauma, in which the pits are shallow and irregular.[6] They uncommonly occur as a

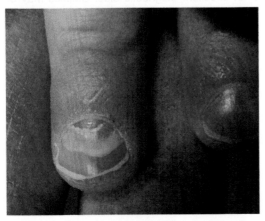

Fig. 11. Onychomadesis in a toddler, resulting from hand-foot-and-mouth syndrome.

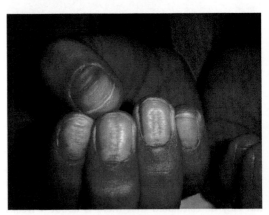

Fig. 13. Habit tic with added longitudinal gutter.

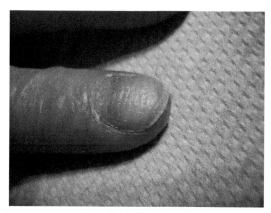

Fig. 14. Pitting in a rippled pattern (psoriasis).

> **Box 1**
> **Principal causes of pitting**
>
> Psoriasis
>
> Atopic dermatitis
>
> Alopecia areata
>
> Physiologic

physiologic variant. Rare causes include lichen planus, Fiessinger-Leroy syndrome, parakeratosis pustulosa, sarcoidosis, and pityriasis rosacea.[1] The main causes for pitting are listed in **Box 1**.

Trachyonychia

The term trachyonychia comes from the Greek τρα χοσ, which means rough. The nail plate shows multiple fine superficial longitudinal ridging, giving the aspect of sandpapered nails.[31] It is caused by a widespread, prolonged, moderate inflammatory process within the proximal matrix.[1] The nail is opaque and shows excessive longitudinal ridging (**Fig. 16**). Thinning of the nail plate causes brittleness, which may be associated with koilonychia and splitting at the free edge (**Fig. 17**). The cuticles are often hyperplastic and ragged. Another type of trachyonychia, called the shiny type, describes surface alterations that are less severe and consist of multiple punctuate depressions that reflect the light. Both types involve 1 or several finger or toenails. The term 20-nail dystrophy has been improperly and widely used for any nail disease affecting the 20 nails or for trachyonychia involving some nails only. It should no longer be used and clinicians now prefer the term trachyonychia. Conditions that may cause trachyonychia include alopecia areata, lichen planus, psoriasis, and eczema. There is no correlation between the clinical features and the cause of trachyonychia. In alopecia areata, trachyonychia is observed in only 12% of cases in children[30] and 3% in adults.[32] The frequency of trachyonychia in psoriasis and lichen planus is not known. The term idiopathic trachyonychia refers to a roughness of 1 or several nail plates without any concomitant skin or hair disease. It remains a rare nail disorder and has been reported mostly in children and men.[33] Tosti and colleagues[34] performed nail biopsies in 23 patients with idiopathic trachyonychia and found spongiotic alterations in 83% of the cases, a psoriatic pattern in 13%, and 4% of the cases were caused by lichen planus. Richert and André[35]

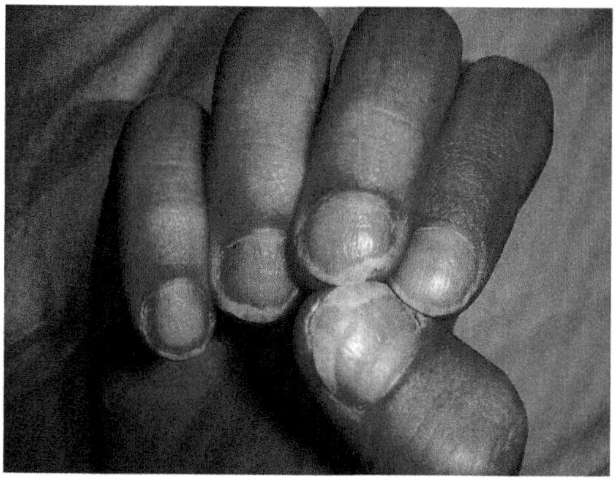

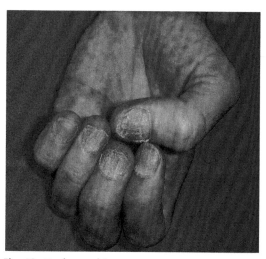

Fig. 15. Shallow pitting in a patient with alopecia areata.

Fig. 16. Trachyonychia.

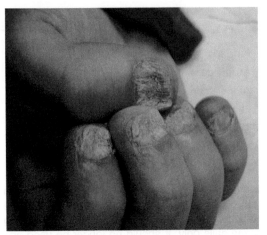

Fig. 17. Severe form of trachyonychia associated with koilonychias from thinning of the plate.

examined 22 cases and found spongiotic changes in 45%, lichen planus in 27%, and psoriasis in 27%.

Trachyonychia associated with clinical alopecia areata usually shows spongiotic alterations but in one case of trachyonychia occurring during alopecia areata histologic examination revealed a lichen planus.[36] Exceptional cases showed that trachyonychia involving the 20 nails was caused by sarcoidosis[37] or pemphigus.[38]

Only a lateral longitudinal biopsy allows the diagnosis to be made. It is not recommended because it is a benign self-limited abnormality that slowly resolves spontaneously with age.[31,39–41] A small series on 12 cases concluded that half of the patients showed total resolution or marked improvement within the first 6 years regardless of treatment.[42] The main causes for trachyonychia are listed in **Box 2**.

Elkonyxis

This is a rare nail surface dystrophy: the nail appears to have been punched out at its most proximal part, mainly in a median position. This deep, narrow, roundish defect moves distally with the nail growth. It corresponds with an acute focal transient insult to the proximal matrix. The main causes are trauma and psoriasis. Other causes include secondary syphilis, Fiessinger-Leroy syndrome, and etretinate.[43] Causes for elkonyxis are listed in **Box 3**.

CLINICAL SIGNS OF DISTAL MATRIX INVOLVEMENT

Distal nail matrix involvement presents with chromonychia. The pathologic process is responsible for a modification of the matrix keratinization (ie, leukonychia), for an inflammation of the matrix (ie, erythronychia), or for an activation or a proliferation of the matrix melanocytes (ie, longitudinal melanonychia).

Leukonychia

Leukonychia refers to a nail with a normal surface that has lost its transparency and looks partially or totally white. These forms can be temporary or permanent depending on the cause. Three types of leukonychias should be differentiated[6]:

1. True leukonychia results from a condition disturbing the distal nail matrix keratinization, resulting in the presence of parakeratotic cells entrapped within the ventral portion of the nail plate (they cannot be eliminated as in pits). The nail appears white as the result of the diffraction of light from the parakeratotic cells preventing visualization of the pink vascular bed. Under the microscope, the keratin fibers are fragmented and irregularly aligned.[44] This discoloration does not disappear with pressure.
2. Apparent leukonychia results from nail bed alterations (ie, half nail and half Muehrcke lines). This type of leukonychia disappears with pressure.
3. Pseudoleukonychia refers to a white discoloration of the nail plate resulting neither from the matrix nor the bed (ie, superficial onychomycosis, granulations of keratin).

Box 2
Causes of trachyonychia
Lichen planus
Psoriasis
Spongiosis within the matrix

Box 3
Causes of elkonyxis
Trauma
Psoriasis
Retinoids
Syphilis

True leukonychia may present under different clinical patterns:

- Punctate leukonychia is the least severe form of true leukonychia and presents as 1-mm to 3-mm solitary or grouped spots, almost exclusively on the fingernails. This common form of leukonychia results from minor trauma to the proximal nail fold and the underlying matrix. It is most commonly observed in the fingernails of children and manual workers (**Fig. 18**). The leukonychia may be preceded by a subungual hematoma leading to subsequent abnormal matrix keratinization. The white dots progress distally with the nail growth, but often disappear during their migration toward the free edge, suggesting that parakeratotic cells are capable of maturing and losing their keratohyalin granules to produce keratin.[6] Their presence is not usually associated with systemic diseases, but they may occur in psoriasis or alopecia areata because of inclusions of parakeratotic cells within the nail plate.

- Transverse leukonychia presents as one or more transverse white opaque lines on the nail plate, paralleling the lunula, separated by normal pink nail. When several nails are affected, the white bands are often located at the same level. The most common cause is trauma: it is frequently observed in the fingernails of women, caused by matrix trauma secondary to manicures. The distance between each line allows clinicians to determine the time between each manicure. Occupational work with repeated tasks may also provoke such transverse white lines (**Fig. 19**).

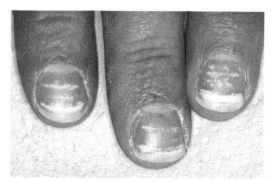

Fig. 19. Transverse leukonychia from repeatedly filing index cards.

Transverse leukonychia on the great toenails from repeated buffeting against the tip of the shoe of an untrimmed nail is also common (**Fig. 20**).[45] In forensic medicine, white transverse bands are a well-known clue for arsenic poisoning.[46,47] Although these bands are named after the Dutch physician Mees,[48] who described the abnormality in 1919, earlier descriptions of the same abnormality had been made by Aldrich[49] from the United States in 1904 and by Reynolds[50] from the United Kingdom in 1901. It is a pity that the term Mees line has not been restricted to arsenic poisoning. Many investigators now call Mees' lines any transverse leukonychia, whatever their origin: thallium intoxication,[51] cyclosporine treatment,[52] chemotherapy[53–56] (especially in children, in whom it is the most common nail change),[54] bacterial infection,[57] parasitic infection,[58] autoimmune diseases,[59] hematologic disorders,[60] or electron beam radiation.[61]

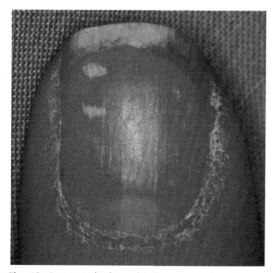

Fig. 18. Punctate leukonychia in a manual worker.

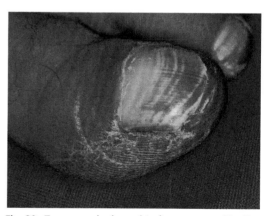

Fig. 20. Transverse leukonychia from repeated buffeting against the tip of the shoe in a woman with abnormal biomechanics of the forefoot.

Table 3
Causes of true leukonychia

Punctuate Leukonychia	Transverse Leukonychia	Longitudinal Leukonychia	Total or Partial Leukonychia
Trauma	Trauma	Darier disease	Congenital
Childhood idiopathic	Heavy metal poisoning	Hailey-Hailey disease	—
Psoriasis	Chemotherapy	Onychopapilloma	—

- Longitudinal leukonychia may be secondary to either nail matrix or nail bed diseases. When originating from the matrix (true leukonychia) it is secondary to a localized metaplasia. It is observed in Darier disease, in which the nail shows longitudinal white lines, red lines, or both at the same time. The white lines correspond with an epithelial hyperplasia of the matrix and the red lines represent a thinned nail from the matrix disease[6]. In Hailey-Hailey disease, longitudinal leukonychia was reported in half of the patients[62] and may be the first clue to the disease. There is no alternation of red and white lines as in Darier disease. Onychopapilloma is a tumor starting in the distal matrix (discussed later). A white variant of onychopapilloma (discussed later) has been reported.[63]

- Total leukonychia is a rare condition. The nail plate is completely opaque and white. It may be milky, chalky, ivory, or porcelain white. Nails with total leukonychia have accelerated growth. The condition may be hereditary and associated with keratoderma and other congenital defects.[6]

The main causes for true leukonychia are listed in **Table 3**.

Erythronychia

Red color in the matrix may present in different ways. A diffuse red color in the lunula (so-called red lunula) may vary from light pink to dark erythema. The color is sharply demarcated and does not extent over the borders of the lunula. This erythema disappears under pressure. Its pathogenesis remains obscure. Red lunula may be encountered in many systemic disorders (**Fig. 21**). Red spots in the lunula (so-called mottled lunula) reflect an acute inflammatory disorder; mainly psoriasis, lichen planus, or alopecia areata (**Fig. 22**). A red longitudinal streak may be observed in 1 or several nails. When the cause is in the matrix, it results from a localized punctate defect in the distal matrix, inducing a longitudinal ventral groove at the undersurface of the nail, which becomes thinner. The nail is more transparent and this permits a better visualization of the vasculature of the nail bed. In addition, the nail bed swells and is trapped in the groove, and the nail bed vessels get engorged, increasing the red color. There is often a keratotic process emerging under the free edge and splinter hemorrhages (**Fig. 23**). This clinical presentation has been called onychopapilloma.[64] Multiple red bands alternating with white bands, on several but not all nails, characterize Darier disease. A

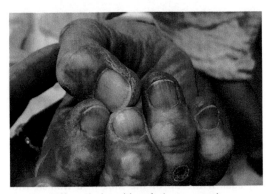

Fig. 21. Diffuse dark red lunula in an argyria.

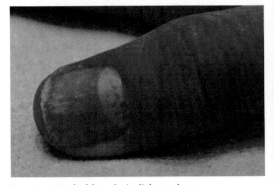

Fig. 22. Mottled lunula in lichen planus.

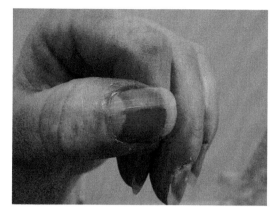

Fig. 23. Onychopapilloma. Note the notch in the distal matrix where the lesion originates.

single painful longitudinal erythronychia, with a distal notch, in a woman in her 40s, is the hallmark of a submatricial glomus tumor. The main causes of erythronychia are listed in **Table 4**.

MELANONYCHIA

Longitudinal melanonychia refers to the presence of melanin within the nail plate and results either from activation of nail matrix melanocytes (friction, drugs) or from melanocyte hyperplasia (lentigo, nevus, and melanoma). Longitudinal melanonychia presents clinically as 1 or more longitudinal pigmented bands extending from the proximal nail fold to the free edge. The band of melanonychia can vary in color and in width. Dermatoscopy of the free edge of the nail allows the level of nail plate pigmentation and its probable origin in the proximal or distal nail matrix to be determined (see **Fig. 1D**).[65]

Table 4 Causes of erythronychia	
Monodactylous single erythronychia	Onychopapilloma Glomus tumor Matricial scar Bowen disease
Monodactylous multiple erythronychia	Hemiplegia
Polydactylous multiple erythronychia	Darier disease
Red lunulae	Systemic diseases

REFERENCES

1. Nicolopoulos J, Goodman GJ, Howard A. Diseases of the generative nail apparatus. Part I: nail matrix. Australas J Dermatol 2002;43:81–90 [quiz: 91–2].
2. André J, Sass U, Richert B, et al. Nail pathology. Clin Dermatol 2013;31:526–39.
3. De Berker D, Wojnarowska F, Sviland L, et al. Keratin expression in the normal nail unit: markers of regional differentiation. Br J Dermatol 2000;142:89–96.
4. Perrin C, Michiels JF, Pisani A, et al. Anatomic distribution of melanocytes in normal nail unit: an immunohistochemical investigation. Am J Dermatopathol 1997;19:462–7.
5. de Berker D. Nail anatomy. Clin Dermatol 2013;31: 509–15.
6. Dawber RP, de Berker DA, Baran R. Science of the nail apparatus. Diseases of the nails and their management. 2nd edition. Oxford (United Kingdom): Blackwell Science; 1994. p. 1–34.
7. Yaemsiri S, Hou N, Slining MM, et al. Growth rate of human fingernails and toenails in healthy American young adults. J Eur Acad Dermatol Venereol 2010; 24:420–3.
8. Dawber R. Fingernail growth in normal and psoriatic subjects. Br J Dermatol 1970;82:454–7.
9. Dawber R, Baran R. Nail growth. Cutis 1987;39: 99–103.
10. Baran R. Pathologie des ongles du sujet âgé. Rev Gen Gérontol 1997;33:43–8.
11. Griego RD, Orengo IF, Scher RK. Median nail dystrophy and habit tic deformity: are they different forms of the same disorder? Int J Dermatol 1995;34: 799–800.
12. Bottomley WW, Cunliffe WJ. Median nail dystrophy associated with isotretinoin therapy. Br J Dermatol 1992;127:447–8.
13. Dharmagunawardena B, Charles-Holmes R. Median canaliform dystrophy following isotretinoin therapy. Br J Dermatol 1997;137:658–9.
14. De Berker D. What do Beau's lines mean? Int J Dermatol 1994;33:545–6.
15. Singh M, Kaur S. Chemotherapy-induced multiple Beau's lines. Int J Dermatol 1986;25:590–1.
16. Wolf D, Wolf R, Goldberg MD. Beau's lines. A case report. Cutis 1982;29:191–4.
17. Guimbao J, Rodrigo P, Alberto MJ, et al. Onychomadesis outbreak linked to hand, foot, and mouth disease, Spain, July 2008. Euro Surveill 2010;15(37).
18. Cabrerizo M, De Miguel T, Armada A, et al. Onychomadesis after a hand, foot, and mouth disease outbreak in Spain, 2009. Epidemiol Infect 2010; 138:1775–8.
19. Wei SH, Huang YP, Liu MC, et al. An outbreak of coxsackievirus A6 hand, foot, and mouth disease associated with onychomadesis in Taiwan, 2010. BMC Infect Dis 2011;11:346.

20. Davia JL, Bel PH, Ninet VZ, et al. Onychomadesis outbreak in Valencia, Spain associated with hand, foot, and mouth disease caused by enteroviruses. Pediatr Dermatol 2011;28:1–5.

21. Bettoli V, Zauli S, Toni G, et al. Onychomadesis following hand, foot, and mouth disease: a case report from Italy and review of the literature. Int J Dermatol 2013;52:728–30.

22. Miyamoto A, Hirata R, Ishimoto K, et al. An outbreak of hand-foot-and-mouth disease mimicking chicken pox, with a frequent association of onychomadesis in Japan in 2009: a new phenotype caused by coxsackievirus A6. Eur J Dermatol 2014;24:103–4.

23. Downing C, Ramirez-Fort MK, Doan HQ, et al. Coxsackievirus A6 associated hand, foot and mouth disease in adults: clinical presentation and review of the literature. J Clin Virol 2014;60:381–6.

24. Macaulay WL. Transverse ridging of the thumbnails. "Washboard thumbnails". Arch Dermatol 1966;93: 421–3.

25. Plinck EP. Diagnostic image. A boy with washboard nails. Ned Tijdschr Geneeskd 2002;146(39):1859–60.

26. Wu JJ. Habit tic deformity secondary to guitar playing. Dermatol Online J 2009;15:16.

27. Lee YB, Cheon MS, Eun YS, et al. Elkonyxis in association with washboard nail and 20-nail dystrophy. Int J Dermatol 2014;53:e11–3.

28. Tham SN, Lim JJ, Tay SH, et al. Clinical observations on nail changes in psoriasis. Ann Acad Med Singap 1988;17:482–5.

29. Al-Mutairi N, Manchanda Y, Nour-Eldin O. Nail changes in childhood psoriasis: a study from Kuwait. Pediatr Dermatol 2007;24:7–10.

30. Tosti A, Morelli R, Bardazzi F, et al. Prevalence of nail abnormalities in children with alopecia areata. Pediatr Dermatol 1994;11:112–5.

31. Hazelrigg DE, Duncan WC, Jarratt M. Twenty-nail dystrophy of childhood. Arch Dermatol 1977;113:73–5.

32. Tosti A, Bardazzi F, Piraccini BM, et al. Is trachyonychia, a variety of alopecia areata, limited to the nails? J Invest Dermatol 1995;104(5 Suppl):27S–8S.

33. Tosti A, Fanti PA, Morelli R, et al. Trachyonychia associated with alopecia areata: a clinical and pathologic study. J Am Acad Dermatol 1991;25(2 Pt 1): 266–70.

34. Tosti A, Bardazzi F, Piraccini BM, et al. Idiopathic trachyonychia (twenty-nail dystrophy): a pathological study of 23 patients. Br J Dermatol 1994;131:866–72.

35. Richert B, André J. Trachyonychia: a clinical and histological study of 22 cases. J Eur Acad Dermatol Venereol 1999;12(Suppl 2):S126.

36. Joshi RK, Abanmi A, Ohman SG, et al. Lichen planus of the nails presenting as trachyonychia. Int J Dermatol 1993;32:54–5.

37. Blanco FP, Scher RK. Trachyonychia: case report and review of the literature. J Drugs Dermatol 2006;5:469–72.

38. Berker DD, Dalziel K, Dawber RP, et al. Pemphigus associated with nail dystrophy. Br J Dermatol 1993;129:461–4.

39. Grover C, Khandpur S, Reddy BS, et al. Longitudinal nail biopsy: utility in 20-nail dystrophy. Dermatol Surg 2003;29:1125–9.

40. Gordon KA, Vega JM, Tosti A. Trachyonychia: a comprehensive review. Indian J Dermatol Venereol Leprol 2011;77:640–5.

41. Sehgal VN. Twenty nail dystrophy trachyonychia: an overview. J Dermatol 2007;34(6):361–6.

42. Sakata S, Howard A, Tosti A, et al. Follow up of 12 patients with trachyonychia. Australas J Dermatol 2006;47:166–8.

43. Cannata GE, Gambetti M. Elconyxis, une complication inconnue de l'étrétinate. Nouv Dermatol 1990;9:251.

44. Laporte M, André J, Achten G. Microscopic approach to true leukonychia. In: Proceedings of the World Congress of Dermatology. London: CRC Press; 1993. p. 375–6.

45. Baran R, Perrin C. Transverse leukonychia of toenails due to repeated microtrauma. Br J Dermatol 1995;133:267–9.

46. Quecedo E, Sanmartin O, Febrer MI, et al. Mees' lines: a clue for the diagnosis of arsenic poisoning. Arch Dermatol 1996;132:349–50.

47. Seavolt MB, Sarro RA, Levin K, et al. Mees' lines in a patient following acute arsenic intoxication. Int J Dermatol 2002;41:399–401.

48. Mees RA. Een verschijnsel bij polyneuritis arsenicosa. Ned Tijdschr Geneeskd 1919;63:391–6.

49. Aldrich CJ. Leuconychia striata arsenicalis transversus, with report of three cases. Am J Med Sci 1904; 127:707–9.

50. Reynolds ES. An account of the epidemic outbreak of arsenical poisoning occurring in beer drinkers in the north of England and the midland countries in 1900. Med Chir Trans 1901;84:409–52.

51. Zhao G, Ding M, Zhang B, et al. Clinical manifestations and management of acute thallium poisoning. Eur Neurol 2008;60:292–7.

52. Siragusa M, Schepis C, Cosentino FI, et al. Nail pathology in patients with hemiplegia. Br J Dermatol 2001;144:557–60.

53. Ceyhan AM, Yildirim M, Bircan HA, et al. Transverse leukonychia (Mees' lines) associated with docetaxel. J Dermatol 2010;37:188–9.

54. Chen W, Yu YS, Liu YH, et al. Nail changes associated with chemotherapy in children. J Eur Acad Dermatol Venereol 2007;21:186–90.

55. Shelley WB, Humphrey GB. Transverse leukonychia (Mees' lines) due to daunorubicin chemotherapy. Pediatr Dermatol 1997;14:144–5.

56. Kim IS, Lee JW, Park KY, et al. Nail change after chemotherapy: simultaneous development of Beau's lines and Mees' lines. Ann Dermatol 2012; 24:238–9.

57. Fujita Y, Sato-Matsumura KC, Doi I, et al. Transverse leukonychia (Mees' lines) associated with pleural empyema. Clin Exp Dermatol 2007;32:127–8.

58. Hepburn MJ, English JC, Meffert JJ. Mees' lines in a patient with multiple parasitic infections. Cutis 1997; 59:321–3.

59. Jarek MJ, Finger DR, Gillil WR, et al. Periorbital edema and Mees' lines in systemic lupus erythematosus. J Clin Rheumatol 1996;2:156–9.

60. Anoun S, Qachouh M, Lamchahab M, et al. Mees' lines in an acute myeloid leukemia patient. Turk J Haematol 2013;30:340.

61. Eros N, Marschalkó M, Bajcsay A, et al. Transient leukonychia after total skin electron beam irradiation. J Eur Acad Dermatol Venereol 2011;25:115–7.

62. Burge SM, Wilkinson JD. Darier-White disease: a review of the clinical features in 163 patients. J Am Acad Dermatol 1992;27:40–50.

63. Criscione V, Telang G, Jellinek NJ. Onychopapilloma presenting as longitudinal leukonychia. J Am Acad Dermatol 2010;63:541–2.

64. Baran R, Perrin C. Longitudinal erythronychia with distal subungual keratosis: onychopapilloma of the nail bed and Bowen's disease. Br J Dermatol 2000;143:132–5.

65. Braun RP, Baran R, Saurat JH, et al. Surgical pearl: dermoscopy of the free edge of the nail to determine the level of nail plate pigmentation and the location of its probable origin in the proximal or distal nail matrix. J Am Acad Dermatol 2006;55:512–3.

Diagnosis Using the Nail Bed and Hyponychium

Dr. Eshini Perera, MBBS, B.MedSci, MMed, MPH[a,b],
Prof. Rodney Sinclair, MBBS, MD, FACD[a,b,c],*

KEYWORDS

- Nail bed • Hyponychium • Onycholysis • Pterygium • Subungual tumors
- Squamous cell carcinoma • Melanoma • Glomus tumor

KEY POINTS

- All 20 nails should be examined carefully.
- Common disorders affecting the nail bed include onycholysis, subungual hyperkeratosis, and ventral pterygium.
- Melanomas, squamous cell carcinoma, Bowen disease, and glomus tumors can also present in the nail bed.
- The ABCDEF guidelines can be used to assess a subungual melanoma.
- A glomus tumor should be considered in patients who present with severe pain triggered by cold.

INTRODUCTION

The nail protects the fingertips and toes. The nail also assists fine motor activities including picking up small items, buttoning clothing, and scratching. Conditions of the nail cause cosmetic concerns, impair fine motor functioning, and affect a patient's quality of life.

Disorders of the nail bed, the area under the nail plate extending from the distal aspect of the lunula to the hyponychium, can cause cosmetic disfigurement, embarrassment, discomfort, or pain. The most common examination findings are onycholysis (separation of the nail plate from the nail bed), subungual hyperkeratosis, and onychogryphosis. Tumors of the nail bed are rare but are often missed because of lack of awareness.

A detailed history can identify or exclude many causes of nail bed disorders. History may focus around the time frame in which the nail changes began; associated skin conditions; preceding trauma to the area; occupation; environmental exposures including nail polish and topical applications; history of recent or chronic illness including diabetes, thyroid dysfunction, and vascular disease; and medications.

PHYSICAL EXAMINATION

All 20 nails should be examined. Nail polish or artificial enhancements should be removed before the examination. Structural changes, color changes, trauma, and infection should be noted. Possible nail bed abnormalities are outlined next.

Onycholysis

The nail, when attached to the underlying nail bed, is transparent. When separate from the nail bed, the air interface makes the nail opaque. Onycholysis refers to the opaque coloration of the nail plate seen with separation of the nail from the underlying nail bed (**Fig. 1**).[1–3] Separation usually occurs as a result of disruption of the distal onychocorneal band.[1–4]

Disclosures: None.
[a] Department of Medicine, Dentistry and Health Sciences, The University of Melbourne, Grattan street, Parkville, Victoria 3010, Australia; [b] Department of Dermatology, Epworth Hospital, Bridge Road, Richmond, Victoria 3121, Australia; [c] Department of Dermatology, Sinclair Dermatology, East Melbourne, Victoria 3002, Australia
* Corresponding author. Department of Dermatology, Sinclair Dermatology, East Melbourne, Victoria 3002, Australia.
E-mail address: rodney.sinclair@sinclairdermatology.com.au

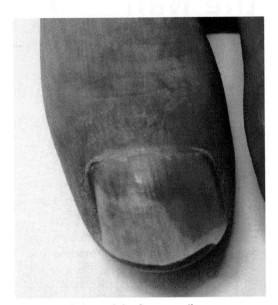

Fig. 1. Onycholysis of the first toenail.

This separation starts at the distal free margin of the nail plate and extends proximally.[1] Stable onycholysis is usually painless and patients often present for cosmetic reasons. Rapid extension of onycholysis, usually the result of minor trauma to the distal free edge of an already onycholytic nail, can be exquisitely painful.

The separation creates a space where secondary infection may occur. In secondary infection the area of separation may present as yellow, brown, or green compared with the white color seen in an uncomplicated onycholysis.

Table 1 outlines some of the causes of onycholysis and their presentations. The most common causes of onycholysis of the toes are trauma or onychomycosis. It is important to examine each toenail separately and to assess the patient's gait. Such clues as the second toe overriding the big toe when shoes are worn and hyperkeratosis of the metatarsal heads or the heel should be noted. The nail bed of a toe that has been traumatized by ill-fitting shoes may

Table 1
Causes of onycholysis

Cause of Onycholysis	Presentation
Onychomycosis	Yellow discoloration Subungual hyperkeratosis and debris Linear spears of onychomycosis extend proximally
Psoriasis	Multiple nails affected Surrounding skin may be red Yellow-brown margin between white area of onycholysis and normal nail Proximal border of the onycholysis is usually irregular Associated nail pitting Onycholysis may begin proximally as a salmon spot (pustular psoriasis of the nail bed)
Trauma	Fingernails usually affected as a result of cleaning underneath the nail with a sharp object Proximal border of onycholysis is usually straight Toenails usually affected by distal trauma from ill-fitting footwear
Infection	*Pseudomonas pyocynae* colonization of the subungual space leads to secondary infection of onycholysis Most common on fingernails
Tumors	Usually only affects one finger Subungual enchondroma or osteoma tents overlying nail leading to distal separation of nail plate from nail bed
Idiopathic	Usually occurs in fingernails
Drugs	Usually occurs in all nails Hemorrhagic changes may be present Thumb may be spared in photo-onycholysis
Lichen planus	Fingernail affected Nail thinning Fissuring of nails Patients need to be examined for oral involvement

Adapted from Daniel CR 3rd, Iorizzo M, Piraccini BM, et al. Simple onycholysis. Cutis 2011;87(5):227; with permission.

present with a blister on the nail bed with onycholysis or with an oozing nail bed. Hyperextension of the great toe during the propulsive phase of the gait is a common cause of footwear trauma to the great toenail. This may lead to either onycholysis or onychogryphosis.

Onycholysis is frequently perpetuated by recurrent injury to the already damaged nail. After treating any recognized precipitating cause, onycholysis is principally managed by protecting the nail from minor trauma. The nail is cut short and straight with the area of onycholysis clipped fortnightly. The patient should be advised to dry the digits carefully after exposure to water and to avoid nail polish until the onycholysis has resolved. The free edge of the nail can be taped to promote adherence to the nail bed. Where possible gloves should be warn to avoid exposing the nail to water. In the case of onycholysis of the toenail, in addition to clipping the nails short, properly fitted shoes with a high toe-box should be worn in place of tight-fitting, narrow-toed, or high heels. A gait assessment by a podiatrist may identify hyperextension of the great toe during the propulsive phase. This can be corrected by orthotics that support the metacarpal heads.

Subungual Hyperkeratosis

Subungual hyperkeratosis is the thickening of the stratum corneum of the nail bed and the accumulation of keratinocytes and debris under the nail plate.[5] The nail bed appears thickened and the nail plate is raised from the nail bed. The nail plate may vary in color from yellow to white depending on the cause. Subungual hyperkeratosis may be hereditary or congenital. The most common causes are fungal infection and psoriasis.[6] In a fungal nail infection subungual hyperkeratosis usually presents with onycholysis. **Table 2** outlines the causes of subungual hyperkeratosis. A scraping can be used to differentiate between tinea unguium, psoriasis, and other causes.

Onychogryphosis

Acquired onychogryphosis most commonly affects the great toenails and presents as a thickened opaque nail on a hyperplastic nail bed. The nail plate lateral curvature is accentuated and the nail narrows distally. It may resemble a ram's horn. Pressure from footwear is the most common cause. Rare causes include psoriasis, poor peripheral circulation, scarring of the nail bed, ichthyosis, pemphigus, and syphilis.

Table 2
Causes of subungual hyperkeratosis and the differentiating clinical features

Cause	Differentiating Clinical Features
Tinea unguium	Onycholysis Usually affects toenails Nail color may appear yellow or brown
Psoriasis	Pitting in nail May have cutaneous or joint manifestation of psoriasis
Chronic eczema	Pitting Transverse ridging/furrows in nails Scaling Erythema
Lichen planus	Ridging of nail Rough nail Pterygium Nail dystrophy
Reiter syndrome	Nails may be reddish brown

Pterygium Inversus Unguis (Ventral Pterygium)

Pterygium inversus unguis (ventral pterygium) is a physical finding where the hyponychium adheres to the underside of the nail plate.[7,8] As the nail plate grows the hyponychium extends forward and the distal nail groove is eliminated (**Fig. 2**). The term pterygium inversus unguis is relatively new, and was first described in 1973.[7] This finding occurs commonly in females.[8] Pterygium inversus

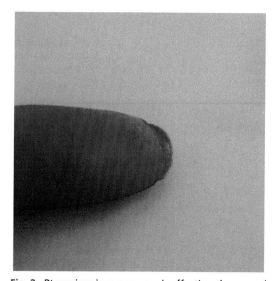

Fig. 2. Pterygium inversus unguis affecting the second finger of the left hand. The hyponychium extends forward as the nail plate grows.

forms are thought to be associated with an abnormality in the development of the nail in the embryo.[11] Causes of a ventral pterygium are listed in **Box 1**.

Currently there are no medical treatments for pterygium inversus unguis; however, gently massaging the area with cuticle creams may help. The hyponychium should not be pushed back because this can cause pain and bleeding. Care should be taken not to cut the hyponychium when trimming the nails. Surgical correction is rarely feasible.

unguis is often acquired; however, some cases may be associated with familial or congenital causes.[9] Acquired forms may occur because of a systemic connective tissue disease or may be idiopathic. Usually more than one nail is affected.

One hypothesis for the development of pterygium inversus unguis is that the pterygium is caused by abnormal circulation, and the scars that develop from ulcerations and healing of the hyponychium result in a loss of the distal nail groove.[10] Congenital

OTHER NAIL BED FINDINGS

Several physical signs can be found in the nail bed. These are associated with a variety of systemic causes. **Table 3** lists some of these nail bed findings and the associated disease.

TUMORS

Several different benign and malignant tumors can affect the nail bed. These are discussed next.

Table 3
Nail bed findings and the associated disease

Nail Bed Finding	Appearance	Cause/Associated Disease
Splinter hemorrhage (Fig. 3)	Vertical red-brown lines of clotted blood Typically look like splinters under the fingernails	Atopic dermatitis Exfoliative dermatitis Lichen planus Onychomycosis Pemphigoid Pemphigus Psoriasis Histiocytosis X Darier disease Infective endocarditis
Terry nail	White ground-glass appearance of the nails on the distal aspect of the nail plate No lunula present	Age: old or young Hereditary Congestive heart failure Pulmonary eosinophilia Liver cirrhosis Ulcerative colitis
Muehrcke lines	White lines running parallel to the lunula Lines run horizontally down the lunula Lines blanch when pressed	Glomerulonephritis Hypoalbuminemia Nephrotic syndrome Acrodermatitis enteropathica Chemotherapy Trauma
White-red longitudinal streaks	—	Darier disease Hailey-Hailey disease Tumor of the nail bed
Oil-drop	Translucent yellow-red colored area Has the appearance of an oil drop	Psoriasis Acroputulosis Systemic lupus erythematosus

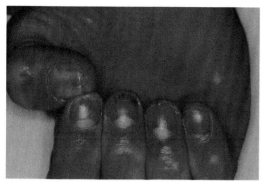

Fig. 3. Splinter hemorrhage affecting the first, second, and third fingernails. (*Courtesy of* Antonella Tosti, MD, Miami, FL.)

Subungual Squamous Cell Carcinomas and Bowen Disease

Squamous cell carcinoma (SCC) and SCC in situ (Bowen disease) are the most common malignant neoplasms of the hand.[12] However, SCC and SCC in situ of the nail apparatus have a low incidence.[13] Known carcinogens include ultraviolet radiation[12] and human papilloma virus (HPV). The role of ultraviolet radiation is likely to be quite minor given the given that ultraviolet A penetrates the nail plate but ultraviolet B cannot. HPV16 and HPV18 have been implicated in genital warts and subungual SCC.[12] In one study, HPV16 DNA was found in roughly 60% of subungual SCC.[12,14] Other factors that may predispose to SCC of the nail apparatus include chronic paronychia, congenital ectodermal dysplasia, and trauma.

Subungual SCC and SCC in situ tend to occur most commonly on the fingernails; however, 16% of cases affect the toenails[15] and 44% of SCC occur on the thumb.[15] Multiple nails may be affected simultaneously.[15]

Subungual SCC in situ can present with subungual erythema, scaling, and distal onycholysis. It may be mistaken for a periungual wart. Pain, swelling of the finger, and inflammation tend to indicate invasive SCC. Advanced cases may present as a chronic discharging ulcer.

Subungual Melanoma

Subungual melanomas are a rare malignancy that arises in the nail matrix, but may extend to involve the nail bed.[16] Subungual melanomas make up 0.7% to 3.5% of cutaneous melanomas.[17–19] The survival rates of subungual melanoma are relatively low because of delayed detection.[16,19] Subungual melanomas occur commonly in patients aged 50 to 70 and occur in all ethnic groups equally.[20] Up to 90% of subungual melanomas

affect the great toe or the thumb.[21] The tumor may present initially with longitudinal melanonychia of a single nail that is wider than 3 mm and expanding proximally. Distal splitting of the nail or nail destruction may occur.[22] Subungual bleeding can also occur.[23] Black discoloration of the proximal or lateral nail fold is known as Hutchinson sign and is considered pathognomic for nail melanoma. Amelanotic subungual melanomas are extremely difficult to diagnose.[24,25] **Table 4** outlines guidelines for subungual melanomas.[16]

Differential diagnoses include subungual hematoma (**Fig. 4**), glomus tumor, subungual SCC, granuloma, benign nevus, or simply normal pigmentation of ethnic skin. Systemic condition, such as vitamin B_{12} or folate deficiency, Cushing disease, and Addison disease, can cause nail pigmentation.[16] Some of these conditions can be distinguished on dermoscopy.[16] Biopsy of the nail should include the nail bed, the matrix, and the nail plate.

Five-year survival rates are 40% for invasive subungual melanomas,[17] with survival inversely related to thickness of the tumor. Treatment is wide local excision for melanoma in situ thin melanoma and amputation for thicker melanoma.

Glomus Tumor

Glomus tumors are benign vascular neoplasms of the glomus body and account for 5.5% of all nail-unit tumors.[26] The glomus body is a neuroarterial structure concentrated in the digits and is thought to have a thermoregulatory function.[27,28] The tumor is usually solitary and predominantly occurs in the nail bed; however, it may manifest in the hand and less frequently other body locations including liver, pancreas, kidneys, and bone.[29–32] Patients present with severe localized tenderness and pain with cold temperatures.[29] Red discoloration of the nail plate over the tumor is common.

Table 4		
ABCDEF guideline for assessing subungual melanomas		
A	Age: occurs between the age of 50 and 70	
B	Brown-black band	
C	Change in size or growth	
D	Digit–thumb, big toe, or index finger usually affected	
E	Extension of color: Hutchinson sign	
F	Family history of melanoma	

From Patel GA, Ragi G, Krysicki J, et al. Subungual melanoma: a deceptive disorder. Acta Dermatovenerol Croat 2008;16(4):239; with permission.

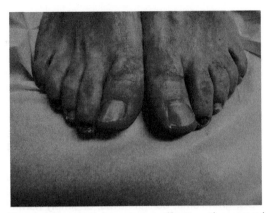

Fig. 4. Subungual hematoma affecting the second and fourth toe of the right foot and the second toe of the left foot. Subungual hematomas may be mistaken for subungual melanomas. (*Courtesy of* Antonella Tosti, MD, Miami, FL.)

Erythronychia and distal onycholysis may be present. Deformity of the nail plate is rare. A plain film, ultrasound, or MRI of the nail helps identify the tumor. An ultrasound can detect glomus tumors from 2 mm in size.[33] Subungual lesions are usually treated by surgical excision with preservation of the nail plate.

SUMMARY

Common conditions of the nail bed include onycholysis, subungual hyperkeratosis, onychogryphosis, ventral pterygium, oil-spots, Terry nails, Muehrcke lines, or splinter hemorrhage. All 20 nails should be examined carefully to look for clues that may point to the cause. Common causes include fungal nail infection, psoriasis, eczema, and lichen planus. Subungual SCC and melanoma can affect the nail bed and diagnostic delays may adversely affects prognosis. Glomus tumors present with localized tenderness or pain made worse with cold.

REFERENCES

1. Daniel CR 3rd, Iorizzo M, Piraccini BM, et al. Simple onycholysis. Cutis 2011;87(5):226–8.
2. Daniel CR 3rd. Onycholysis: an overview. Semin Dermatol 1991;10(1):34–40.
3. Daniel CR 3rd, Daniel MP, Daniel CM, et al. Chronic paronychia and onycholysis: a thirteen-year experience. Cutis 1996;58(6):397–401.
4. Kechijian P. Onycholysis of the fingernails: evaluation and management. J Am Acad Dermatol 1985; 12(3):552–60.
5. Baran R, Haneke E. The nail in differential diagnosis. London: CRC Press; 2006.
6. Nagar R, Nayak CS, Deshpande S, et al. Subungual hyperkeratosis nail biopsy: a better diagnostic tool for onychomycosis. Indian J Dermatol Venereol Leprol 2012;78(5):620–4.
7. Caputo R, Prandi G. Pterygium inversum unguis. Arch Dermatol 1973;108(6):817–8.
8. Caputo R, Cappio F, Rigoni C, et al. Pterygium inversum unguis. Report of 19 cases and review of the literature. Arch Dermatol 1993;129(10):1307–9.
9. Richert BJ, Patki A, Baran R. Pterygium of the nail. Cutis 2000;66:343–6.
10. Patterson JW. Pterygium inversum unguis-like changes in scleroderma. Report of four cases. Arch Dermatol 1977;113(10):1429–30.
11. Odom RB, Stein KM, Maibach HI. Congenital, painful, aberrant hyponychium. Arch Dermatol 1974; 110(1):89–90.
12. Zabawski EJ Jr, Washak RV, Cohen JB, et al. Squamous cell carcinoma of the nail bed: is finger predominance another clue to etiology? A report of 5 cases. Cutis 2001;67(1):59–64.
13. Schiavon M, Mazzoleni F, Chiarelli A, et al. Squamous cell carcinoma of the hand: fifty-five case reports. J Hand Surg Am 1988;13(3):401–4.
14. Moy RL, Eliezri YD, Nuovo GJ, et al. Human papillomavirus type 16 DNA in periungual squamous cell carcinomas. JAMA 1989;261(18):2669–73.
15. Guitart J, Bergfeld WF, Tuthill RJ, et al. Squamous cell carcinoma of the nail bed: a clinicopathological study of 12 cases. Br J Dermatol 1990; 123(2):215–22.
16. Patel GA, Ragi G, Krysicki J, et al. Subungual melanoma: a deceptive disorder. Acta Dermatovenerol Croat 2008;16(4):236–42.
17. Dasgupta T, Brasfield R. Subungual melanoma: 25-year review of cases. Ann Surg 1965;161:545–52.
18. Shaw JH, Koea JB. Acral (volar-subungual) melanoma in Auckland, New Zealand. Br J Surg 1988; 75(1):69–72.
19. Levit EK, Kagen MH, Scher RK, et al. The ABC rule for clinical detection of subungual melanoma. J Am Acad Dermatol 2000;42(2 Pt 1):269–74.
20. Tan KB, Moncrieff M, Thompson JF, et al. Subungual melanoma: a study of 124 cases highlighting features of early lesions, potential pitfalls in diagnosis, and guidelines for histologic reporting. Am J Surg Pathol 2007;31(12):1902–12.
21. Cohen PJ, Hofmann MA, Sterry W, et al. Melanoma. In: Schwartz RA, editor. Skin cancer recognition and management. 2nd edition. Oxford (United Kingdom): Blackwell Publishing; 2008. p. 152–99.
22. Takematsu H, Obata M, Tomita Y, et al. Subungual melanoma. A clinicopathologic study of 16 Japanese cases. Cancer 1985;55(11):2725–31.
23. Thomas L, Dalle S. Dermoscopy provides useful information for the management of melanonychia striata. Dermatol Ther 2007;20(1):3–10.

24. Briggs JC. Subungual malignant melanoma: a review article. Br J Plast Surg 1985;38(2):174–6.

25. Hudson DA, Krige JE, Strover RM, et al. Subungual melanoma of the hand. J Hand Surg Br 1990;15(3):288–90.

26. Girisha BS, Shenoy MM, Mathias M, et al. Glomus tumor of the nail unit. Indian J Dermatol 2011;56(5):583–4.

27. Fujioka H, Kokubu T, Akisue T, et al. Treatment of subungual glomus tumor. Kobe J Med Sci 2009;55(1):E1–4.

28. Drape JL, Idy-Peretti I, Goettmann S, et al. Standard and high resolution magnetic resonance imaging of glomus tumors of toes and fingertips. J Am Acad Dermatol 1996;35(4):550–5.

29. Kim DH. Glomus tumor of the finger tip and MRI appearance. Iowa Orthop J 1999;19:136–8.

30. Miliauskas JR, Worthley C, Allen PW. Glomangiomyoma (glomus tumour) of the pancreas: a case report. Pathology 2002;34(2):193–5.

31. Al-Ahmadie HA, Yilmaz A, Olgac S, et al. Glomus tumor of the kidney: a report of 3 cases involving renal parenchyma and review of the literature. Am J Surg Pathol 2007;31(4):585–91.

32. Simmons TJ, Bassler TJ, Schwinn CP, et al. Case report 749: primary glomus tumor of bone. Skeletal Radiol 1992;21(6):407–9.

33. Marchadier A, Cohen M, Legre R. Subungual glomus tumors of the fingers: ultrasound diagnosis. Chir Main 2006;25(1):16–21.

Nail Surgery
Best Way to Obtain Effective Anesthesia

Nathaniel J. Jellinek, MD[a,b,c],*, Nicole F. Vélez, MD[a]

KEYWORDS

- Nail surgery • Nail biopsy • Dermatologic surgery • Nail biopsy • Digital anesthesia
- Anesthesia of the nail unit • Anesthesia complications

KEY POINTS

- Anesthesia of the nail unit requires a complete understanding of the anatomic and physiologic pathways of pain and the different anesthetic choices.
- Buffering and warming the local anesthetic coupled with a slow rate of injection and small needle size, all drastically reduce pain of injection.
- Local infiltrative anesthesia, termed a wing block, is an efficient and well-tolerated form of anesthesia; however, proper performance uses distracting anesthesia and slow rate of injection.
- Traditional digital block involves injections at the base/sides of the digit and allowance of time for anesthesia to take effect.
- Single-digit injection techniques (transthecal) are effective on the second to fourth fingers and provide complete anesthesia; however, postoperative pain may be more than with other techniques.

 Videos of infiltrative anesthesia and nerve blockade of the bilateral dorsal/volar digital nerves accompany this article at http://www.derm.theclinics.com/

INTRODUCTION, TREATMENT GOALS, AND PLANNED OUTCOMES

Successful nail surgery requires complete anesthesia. Sometimes it is this initial step in nail surgery that most intimidates the patient and, quite often, the physician. As such, mastery of digital anesthesia is a prerequisite to performing competent surgery on the nail apparatus. Administering digital anesthesia requires a multifaceted understanding of the anatomy of the digit, pathophysiology of pain, mechanisms of local anesthetics, and nuances in both technique and preparation that maximize effectiveness of the procedure.

Digital nerves run along each digit as paired parallel volar and dorsal nerves, terminating just beyond the distal interphalangeal joint (DIPJ), where they divide into 3 branches, supplying the nail bed, the digital tip, and pulp.[1] There is no clear consensus on which specific branches innervate the tips for each digit. Generally accepted dogma is that the second to fourth fingertips are innervated by the volar branches, whereas the thumb

Conflicts of Interest: None.
Funding Sources: None.
Prior Presentation: None.

[a] Dermatology Professionals, Inc, 1672 South County Trail, East Greenwich, RI 02818, USA; [b] Division of Dermatology, University of Massachusetts Medical School, Worcester, MA 01655, USA; [c] Department of Dermatology, The Warren Alpert Medical School at Brown University, Providence, RI 02903, USA
* Corresponding author. 1672 South County Trail, Suite 101, East Greenwich, RI 02818.
E-mail address: winenut15@yahoo.com

Dermatol Clin 33 (2015) 265–271
http://dx.doi.org/10.1016/j.det.2014.12.007

and fifth fingertips are innervated primarily by the dorsal branches. These sensory nerves carry the impulses from the many smaller nociceptors located in the nail unit and surrounding tissue to the brain.

Cutaneous nociceptors provide an innate protective warning system for injury and consist of Pacinian corpuscles (movement-sensitive hair follicle receptors), Ruffini corpuscles (pressure sensitive mechanoreceptors), and free-ended nociceptors located at the dermoepidermal junction.[2,3] There are 2 main classes of nerve fibers—fast/myelinated (A-δ, carrying sharp pain) and slow/unmyelinated (C, carrying dull pain), which are activated by these receptors and transfer impulses of pain. Local anesthetics work by blocking the free nerve endings' voltage-gated sodium channels and nerve depolarization, thus impeding transmission of pain. However, local anesthetics must first diffuse into the nerve cells through hydrophobic cell membranes.

During anesthesia, patients experience pain from 2 distinct and unrelated procedures—the needle insertion and fluid infiltration. The former activates Pacinian corpuscles and mechanoreceptors, which transmit via A-δ fibers to evoke the pinprick sensation, whereas the latter (through chemical irritation and rapid distention of tissue) activates mostly free-ending nociceptors and produces a more intense and continuous pain. Infiltrative anesthesia results from anesthesia of the smallest nerve fibers and blocking initial transmission of nociception, whereas nerve blocks affect larger, usually more proximal nerve fibers and require longer time of onset to diffuse into the nerves and block depolarization.

PREOPERATIVE PLANNING AND PREPARATION, PATIENT POSITIONING, "BEST WAY TO PERFORM"

Several factors may impact the patient's degree of pain from anesthesia and their postoperative discomfort. These factors include both specific characteristics of the anesthetic (molecular composition, pH, temperature, addition of epinephrine) and choice of syringe and needle size, distracting stimuli, and technique of injection. Each of these considerations is highlighted individually below.

Three main anesthetics are used in digital anesthesia—lidocaine, bupivacaine, and ropivacaine (Tables 1 and 2). Lidocaine is still the most widely used and has an unparalleled safety history. It is estimated that more than 300 million doses of lidocaine with epinephrine are injected in dental offices alone each year in the United States. Lidocaine is characterized by quick absorption and near instantaneous anesthesia of the minute nociceptors in the skin. The onset is faster (<1–3 min) than that of either ropivacaine (4.5 min) or bupivacaine (4+ min), with a significantly shorter duration of action (60–120 min). Bupivacaine has a longer onset of action and a longer duration of action (480 min).[2] Ironically, a combination of lidocaine and bupivacaine has not reliably shown superiority over each agent alone. Ropivacaine represents perhaps the current ideal in terms of anesthetic, with a short onset of action, prolonged duration of action (up to 20 hours) and less cardiotoxicity than bupivacaine.[1] In addition, ropivacaine has demonstrated some degree of inherent vasoconstriction (as opposed to the vasodilating effect of lidocaine), with potential benefits of providing a bloodless field.[4,5] A down side to consider with the longer acting anesthetics is the risk of masking pain associated with postoperative complications, including compartment syndrome, infection, and ischemia.[6]

Although there remains misunderstanding about the appropriateness of injecting standard concentrations (1:100,000–1:400,000) of epinephrine with local anesthetic into digits, it is quite clear that in the absence of contraindications (ie, thromboangiitis obliterans, severe peripheral vascular disease, Raynaud disease/phenomenon, or other vasospastic disease), it is safe practice and does

| Table 1 | | | | | |
| Common anesthetics in nail surgery | | | | | |
Anesthetic	Onset (min)	pKa	Duration Without Epinephrine	Duration with Epinephrine	Benefits
Lidocaine	<1	7.7	30–120	60–400	Near instantaneous onset
Bupivacaine	2–5	8.1	120–240	240–480	Longer duration
Ropivacaine	1–15	8.2	120–360	Not defined	Longer duration, Potential vasoconstrictive effects

Abbreviation: pKa, pretty standard.
Adapted from Soriano T, Beynet DP. Anesthesia and analgesia. In: Robinson JK, Hanke CW, Siegel DM, et al, editors. Surgery of the skin, 2nd edition. New York: Elsevier; 2010. p. 45; with permission.

Table 2
Digital anesthesia techniques

	Technique	Considerations	Pros	Cons
Infiltrative				
Wing Block	Inject wheal (0.1–0.2 ml) in proximal nail fold and then inject slowly toward each lateral nail fold to digital tip.	Avoid rapid tissue distention. Most anesthesia should be on dorsal aspect of digit.	Near instantaneous anesthesia. Hemostasis from tissue tamponade.	Discomfort without distracting stimuli or with overzealous injection. Potential for tissue tourniquet if too much fluid injected into pulp.
Nerve Blocks				
TDB	Insert needle into the web space at the level of MCP/MTP joint and inject into the subcutaneous tissue.	During delay of anesthesia, consider soaking digit in chlorhexidine and water.	More complete anesthesia of entire digit. More prolonged anesthesia.	Not instantaneous. Requires (at least) 2 needle punctures. May still require infiltrative anesthesia.
TTB	Insert needle in to the palmar digital creased to bone and inject on pullback, as needle tip exits tendon (within tendon sheath).	Requires 3 ml of anesthesia. Can also inject in same location subcutaneously followed by massage (modified subcutaneous technique).	Single injection	Potentially more postoperative pain at injection site.

Abbreviation: MTP, metatarsophalangeal.

not risk permanent ischemia or digital infarction.[7,8] Epinephrine's positive effects are 2-fold: prolonged anesthetic effect/postoperative analgesia[9] and vasoconstriction to decrease bleeding. The former is much more significant than the latter, as most digital surgeries do not require lengthy anesthesia, and alternative safe options exist to create a bloodless field. In particular, a tourniquet produces an immediate bloodless field, and its removal facilitates rapid, observable reperfusion of the digit postoperatively, without the risk of rare vasospastic complications.[8,10]

Lidocaine, 1%, either plain (pH 6.09) or premixed with epinephrine (pH 4.24), is significantly more acidic than physiologic pH. Indeed, lidocaine with epinephrine is approximately 1000 times more acidic than normal subcutaneous tissue. Injection of this acidic solution is predictably painful. Buffering to physiologic pH can be performed simply by adding 1 to 1.8 ml of 8.4% sodium bicarbonate to 10 ml of lidocaine premixed with epinephrine, producing a mixture with a near physiologic pH.[11–13] This practice has been supported by a recent Cochrane review and meta-analysis.[14,15] Not only is the neutral pH solution less painful during injection, but it also facilitates more efficient anesthesia. At physiologic pH, more lidocaine molecules exist in a unionized state, accelerating passage through the lipophilic cell membranes and allowing for faster onset of action.

Of note, commercial premixed lidocaine with epinephrine is acidic in part to prolong its shelf life and stability. When buffered to physiologic pH, the epinephrine is volatile and does not maintain a uniform concentration over time, whereas there is no effect on the anesthetic efficacy of the lidocaine. To ensure the vasoconstrictive properties of a premixed solution, buffering should be performed immediately before its use.

An underutilized technique for minimizing pain of anesthesia is warming the fluid. Hogan, and colleagues[16] recently published a review and meta-analysis showing that warming anesthetic fluid reduced pain of injection of both buffered and unbuffered anesthetic. Although the head-to-head benefit of warming the anesthetic appears to be less than that of buffering to neutral pH, the combination of both techniques consistently provides the least painful injection without loss of efficacy or duration of action.

Nearly all digital anesthesia is performed in "high resistance" tissues, so that Luer lock syringes are mandatory, and use of the finest point needles (preferably 30 gauge for all injections) is recommended. The small needle decreases pain from puncture and limits the flow of anesthetic infusion, further reducing discomfort from rapid tissue distention. It has been stated that the physician may routinely spend more time prepping the surgical site and administering anesthetic than performing the procedure itself.[1]

The physician may further minimize pain with distraction—psychological (eg, conversation, talking—"talkesthesia," joking) and tactile. The authors have found that playing music, even singing to patients, further distracts patients during anesthesia. Introducing a strong, distinct, physical stimulus near the site of injection through use of a massager (Fig. 1), pinching or tapping the skin, or cooling the skin with a refrigerant spray (Videos 1 and 2) can decrease pain by creating sensory noise and via the gate theory close or narrow the pathways of pain.[12] For those most anxious before injection, administering a fast-acting benzodiazepine orally (midazolam, alprazolam, or diazepam) can considerably reduce the fear of injection.[17] The potential retrograde amnestic effect is an added benefit that may reduce any perceived trauma from the experience.

TECHNIQUES OF INJECTION

There are 2 categories of digital anesthesia—infiltrative and nerve blocks. Infiltrative anesthesia is most useful for routine nail surgery with nearly instantaneous anesthetic effect and without risk of pain from or injury to the proximal digit, nerves, or vessels.

Nerve blocks can be divided into traditional digital block (TDB), with (at least) 2 injections at the base of the digit, or single injection techniques into the palmar-digital crease, either subcutaneous or traditional transthecal (TTB). There are predictable delays between injection and onset of anesthesia, given the need for anesthesia to diffuse into the larger nerves and block depolarization and nerve transmission back from the distal digit to the brain.

Wing Block

Infiltrative anesthesia is typically performed as a wing block for nail surgery, referring to the shape of anesthetic effect as it travels down the lateral nail folds (see Video 1).[18] In this technique, the anesthetic is injected first into the proximal nail fold, approximately halfway between the DIPJ and cuticle. The surgeon can inject 0.1 to 0.2 ml as a wheal, slowly into the nail fold dermis (taking care not to inject too deeply into the matrix.) This injection is followed by gradual, deliberate pressure on the syringe (often significant resistance is encountered), and a gentle fluid bolus is advanced *ahead* of the needle, moving obliquely toward each lateral nail fold, then down the lateral nail folds to the digital tip. When this is performed correctly, the second, third, and subsequent needle insertions are placed into already anesthetized skin, so that only one pinprick is experienced. The anesthetic fluid must be injected slowly to avoid rapid tissue distention. Once the fluid is injected, the digital tip will look white because of fluid load, even with use of plain anesthetic (Fig. 2). Care must be taken not to fill the entire pulp with anesthetic fluid and limit most anesthesia to the dorsal 50% of the digit. The pulp, unlike the nail folds, represents a potential reservoir for several milliliters of fluid. Infiltrating the entire tip, pulp, and periungual tissues with anesthetic—which can accommodate 5 ml or more—can serve as a fluid tourniquet and is not recommended nor necessary for surgery on the nail. When performed properly, infiltrative wing block anesthesia is well tolerated and produces nearly instantaneous and complete nail unit anesthesia and a degree of hemostasis from direct anesthetic tamponade of the nail unit (see Video 1).

Traditional Digital Block

The TDB is still widely used, despite some inherent disadvantages when compared with the infiltrative wing block and single injection technique (see

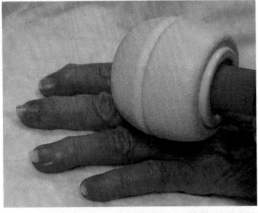

Fig. 1. A vibrating head massager is placed over the proximal digit before and during injection of anesthesia. The closer the placement of the distracting stimulus to the injection, the more robust the benefit.

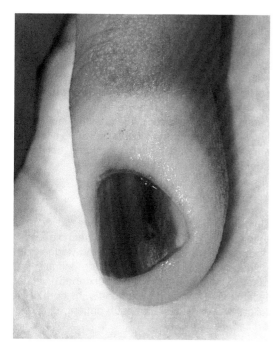

Fig. 2. Immediately after injection of an infiltrative wing block with lidocaine 1% without epinephrine. The tissue is white from fluid bolus (rather than epinephrine-induced vasoconstriction) and limited primarily to the dorsal 50% of the digit.

Video 2). Its efficacy, benefits, and proven safety profile, however, have supported its continued and widespread use. This technique is performed by inserting the needle into the web space at the level of the metacarpophalangeal (MCP) or meta-tarsophalangeal joint from a dorsal to palmar/plantar direction on both sides of the digit (at least 2 separate needle punctures) and injecting the anesthetic into the subcutaneous tissue. Variations exist whereby the anesthesia is injected into the digital sides of the middle phalanx rather than proximally at the MCP joint. In all cases, this type of nerve block anesthetizes the paired dorsal and volar digital nerves. Occasionally, the digital nerves of the adjacent fingers may become anesthetized as well.

There are 2 approaches to the level of needle insertion. Some prefer to insert the needle until it hits the bone, then withdraw a few millimeters and inject in the supraperiosteal plane at the level of the digital nerves. This method provides the most efficient plane of injection but risks needling the nerve itself or adjacent blood vessels.[19] Others, including the authors, prefer to use a more superficial subcutaneous plane of injection. The authors inject a small wheal for initial anesthesia followed by subsequent slow injections angled dorsally and toward the palmar/plantar

direction, with massage of the anesthetic down to the level of the nerves (see Video 2). The patient is then left to wait while the anesthetic diffuses into the nerves. This delay may be as short as 3 minutes[5,6] and as long as 15 to 20 minutes. The surgeon may have the patient soak his or her digit in warm water and chlorhexidine in the meanwhile to soften the nail plate and provide a superficial degree of antisepsis.

With this and all blocks, it is important to check the distal digit and nail unit for complete anesthesia before initiating the procedure; occasionally there may be pockets of unanaesthetized skin distal to the block, requiring either local infiltrative block or additional time for nerve blockade.

Palmar Single-Injection Techniques

Two well-described single injection techniques produce a digital block—the transthecal (traditional or modified approach) block or the related subcutaneous variation. Both work most predictably on the long fingers (second to fourth), supporting the dogma of dominant volar (more than dorsal) digital nerves in the long fingers. The TTB is performed by supinating the hand and inserting the needle perpendicularly into the palmar-digital crease, extending (through flexor tendon and tendon sheath) to bone, then slowly withdrawing the needle while applying gentle pressure to the syringe plunger (**Fig. 3**). As the needle tip exits the tendon during pullback, there is loss of resistance (in the tendon sheath), and the anesthesia is injected slowly into this space, which then diffuses laterally to the digital nerves. Three milliliters of anesthesia are injected, providing quicker onset and lengthier anesthesia than 2 ml.[20]

The subcutaneous technique involves injection of the same volume at the same landmark (ie, one injection) but without deep penetration through the tendon sheath. As described for the TTB above, the anesthetic is slowly injected into the low-resistance subcutaneous plane, and firmly massaged into the deep tissues to facilitate diffusion and anesthesia of the digital nerves. Theoretically, there is less risk of tendon inflammation, injury, or infection with this more superficial plane of injection.

Several studies evaluated the relative advantages and disadvantages of these techniques and compared them in head-to-head studies. There is some evidence for less pain with the TDB and subcutaneous injection versus the TTB.[21,22] The onset of action is fairly similar for all techniques, and the slight differences should not favor one technique over another. Instead, the surgeon's approach should depend on the

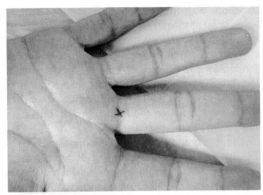

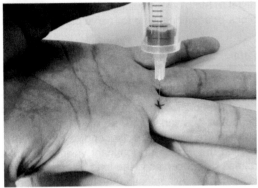

Fig. 3. (*Top*) Digital palmar crease marked with X. (*Bottom*) thirty-gauge needle on Luer lock syringe is inserted perpendicular to the digit with the hand supinated.

particular circumstances of each case, including his or her comfort level, the patient's anxiety regarding the number of needle sticks, and the specific digit involved. Comfort with all of them, however, will allow the most appropriate choice in any given clinical situation.

POTENTIAL COMPLICATIONS AND THEIR MANAGEMENT; POSTPROCEDURAL CARE

Digital anesthesia for nail surgery is remarkably well tolerated. Complications are rare. Prolonged ischemia after injection of epinephrine is most likely in patients with vasospastic disease, as noted previously. Reversal is best performed with locally injected phentolamine, although some report use of nitroglycerine topically. Wing block has been associated with focal superficial necrosis in exceptional cases only.[1] TDB risks injury of needling or injection into the proximal digital nerves or vessels when injected deep just above the bone. Such complications are avoided with more superficial injection, as discussed previously. With the traditional TTB, there is a theoretic risk of tendon sheath infection, tendon rupture, or late occurrence of trigger finger, although to our

knowledge there are no reported cases.[1] The traditional and modified TTB both have shown more prolonged localized pain after anesthesia at the site of injection than other procedures. This pain, however, is transient and nearly always resolves within 1 to 2 days. With all nerve blocks, it is important to recognize the required delay between injection and complete anesthesia. The unknowing surgeon may continue to inject local anesthesia, risking a fluid tourniquet or painful edema of the surgical site.[1,5]

SUMMARY

Complete anesthesia is a prerequisite for successful digital and nail surgery. Several techniques are both effective and well tolerated. Knowledge of the pain pathways, use of distracting stimuli, and mastery of the anatomy and described injection techniques provide the surgeon with comfort to tailor local anesthesia for each patient, digit, and procedure.

SUPPLEMENTARY DATA

Supplementary data related to this article can be found online at http://dx.doi.org/10.1016/j.det. 2014.12.007.

REFERENCES

1. Richert B. Anesthesia of the nail apparatus. In: Richert B, Di Chiacchio N, Haneke E, editors. Nail surgery. New York: Informa Healthcare; 2010. p. 24–30.
2. Soriano T, Beynet DP. Anesthesia and analgesia. In: Robinson JK, Hanke CW, Siegel DM, et al, editors. Surgery of the skin. 2nd edition. New York: Elsevier; 2010. p. 43–63.
3. Egekvist H, Bjerring P, Arendt-Nielsen L. Pain and mechanical injury of human skin following needle insertions. Eur J Pain 1999;3(1):41–9.
4. Keramidas EG, Rodopoulou SG. Ropivacaine versus lidocaine blocks: a prospective study. Plast Reconstr Surg 2007;119:2148–52.
5. Alhelail M, Al-Salamah M, Al-Mulhim M, et al. Comparison of bupivacaine and lidocaine with epinephrine for digital nerve blocks. Emerg Med J 2009; 26:347–50.
6. Vinycomb TI, Sahhar LJ. Comparison of local anesthetics for digital nerve blocks: a systematic review. J Hand Surg Am 2014;39(4):744–51.
7. Harness NG. Digital block anesthesia. J Hand Surg Am 2009;34(1):142–5.
8. Andrade A, Here HG. Traumatic hand injuries: the emergency clinician's evidence-based approach. Emerg Med Pract 2011;13(6):1–24.

9. Schnabi SM, Unglaub F, Leitz Z, et al. Skin perfusion and pain evaluation with different local anaesthetics in a double blind randomized study following digital nerve block anaesthesia. Clin Hemorheol Microcirc 2013;55(2):241–53.

10. Jellinek NJ. Commentary: how much is too much? Tourniquets and digital ischemia. Dermatol Surg 2013;39(4):593–5.

11. Strazar R, Lalonde D. Minimizing injection pain in local anesthesia. CMAJ 2012;184(18):2016.

12. Strazar AR, Leynes PG, Lalonde DH. Minimizing the pain of local anesthesia injection. Plast Reconstr Surg 2013;132(3):675–84.

13. Frank SG, Lalonde DH. How acidic is the lidocaine we are injecting, and how much bicarbonate show we add? Can J Plast Surg 2012;20(2):71–3.

14. Cepeda MS, Tzortzopoulou A, Thackrey M, et al. Adjusting the pH of lidocaine for reducing pain on injection. Cochrane Database Syst Rev 2010;(12):CD006581.

15. Burns CA, Ferris G, Feng C, et al. Decreasing the pain of local anesthesia: a prospective, double-blind comparison of buffered, premixed 1% lidocaine with epinephrine versus 1% lidocaine freshly mixed with epinephrine. J Am Acad Dermatol 2006;54(1):128–31.

16. Hogan ME, vanderVaart S, Perampaladas K, et al. Systematic review and meta-analysis of the effect of warming local anesthetics on injection pain. Ann Emerg Med 2011;58(1):86–98.

17. Ravitskiy L, Phillips PK, Roegnigk RK, et al. The use of oral midazolam for perioperative anxiolysis of healthy patients undergoing Mohs surgery: conclusions from randomized controlled and prospective studies. J Am Acad Dermatol 2011;64(2):310–22.

18. Jellinek NJ. Nail surgery: practical tips and treatment options. Dermatol Ther 2007;20(1):68–74.

19. Cummings AJ, Tisol WB, Meyer LE. Modified transthecal digital block versus traditional digital block for anesthesia of the finger. J Hand Surg Am 2004; 29(1):44–8.

20. Waitayawinyu T, Dodds SD, Niempoog S. Dose effectiveness of transthecal digital block. J Hand Surg Am 2009;34(3):458–62.

21. Keramidas EG, Rodopoulou SG, Tsoutsos D, et al. Comparison of transthecal digital block and traditional digital block for anesthesia of the finger. Plast Reconstr Surg 2004;114(5):1131–4.

22. Yin ZG, Zhang JB, Kan SL, et al. A comparison of traditional digital blocks and single subcutaneous palmar injection blocks at the base of the finger and a meta-analysis of the digital block trials. J Hand Surg Br 2006;31(5):547–55.

Best Way to Perform a Punch Biopsy

Judith Domínguez-Cherit, MD[a],*, Daniela Gutiérrez Mendoza, MD[b]

KEYWORDS

- Nails • Nail punch biopsy • Punch biopsy • Nail surgery • Matrix • Nail bed • Nail plate
- Periungueal folds

KEY POINTS

- Punch biopsy is useful for the diagnosis and treatment of nail diseases.
- The goal of a punch biopsy is to obtain a 2- to 3-mm tissue sample for successful interpretation of nail diseases.
- All anatomic sites of the nail apparatus may be sampled with a punch biopsy.
- It is helpful to soften the nail before the procedure by soaking it in water for 5 minutes.
- Punch biopsy is a simple procedure with rapid healing time and few complications.

 A video of nail punch biopsy accompanies this article at http://www.derm.theclinics.com/

INTRODUCTION

Nail biopsy is used for the diagnosis and treatment of nail diseases. Punch biopsy is among the many techniques that may be used and, like all nail procedures, best results are possible when the surgeon is familiar with the anatomy and the physiology of the nail apparatus.

TREATMENT GOALS AND PLANNED OUTCOMES

The goal of a punch biopsy is to obtain a 2- to 3-mm tissue sample for the diagnosis of nail diseases, to improve a medical condition, or to completely remove a nail tumor.

PREOPERATIVE PLANNING AND PREPARATION

Before performing the procedure, the surgeon must plan the objective of the surgery. If the biopsy is for diagnostic purposes, enough specimen for histologic analysis must be obtained. It must also be handled with care. Often, the tissue obtained from a punch biopsy is difficult to interpret because it is too small and fragile, and becomes damaged during handling.[1]

A second issue to consider is that an experienced surgeon who is familiar with the anatomy and the physiology of the nail apparatus is required to ensure the desired anatomic site is excised and to avoid damage of the area that will lead to postoperative complications. If the goal is to completely remove a lesion that is larger than 3 mm, it is better to consider using another method instead.

It is always helpful to soak the nail in warm water for 5 to 10 minutes before the procedure to soften the nail especially in the case of thick toenails. The entire finger or toe should be cleaned with chlorhexidine or other surgical soap.[2]

No disclosures.

[a] Department of Dermatology, Insituto Nacional de Ciencias Médicas y Nutrición "Salvador Zubiran", Av. Vasco de Quiroga #15, Colonia Belisario Dominguez Sección XVI, Delegación Tlalpan, CP 14000, México Distrito Federal 14000, Mexico; [b] Department of Dermatology, Hospital General "Dr Manuel Gea González", Av. Calzada de Tlalpan #4800, Tlalpan Seccion XVI, CP 14080, México Distrito Federal, Mexico
* Corresponding author.
E-mail addresses: judom59@hotmail.com; dominguez.judith@gmail.com

Dermatol Clin 33 (2015) 273–276
http://dx.doi.org/10.1016/j.det.2014.12.008
0733-8635/15/$ – see front matter © 2015 Elsevier Inc. All rights reserved.

PATIENT POSITIONING

The patient has to be in a comfortable sitting position. To achieve stability, it is best to use an armrest for fingernail procedures. In the case of toenails, a more stable position is attained with a bended knee.

THE BEST WAY TO PERFORM A PUNCH BIOPSY

The following materials are necessary for a punch biopsy:

1. A disposable punch no. 2 or 3;
2. Iris scissors;
3. Suture scissors when necessary;
4. Nail holder; and
5. Cyanoacrylate when necessary.

Fine instruments, like Castroviejo scissors, a nail holder, and forceps are recommended.

THE PROCEDURE

This procedure needs to be done under local anesthesia (Video 1). The proximal nerve block is preferred. In the absence of nail plate, this is the best way to perform a punch biopsy.

1. The disposable punch is positioned vertically, at a 90° angle, or perpendicular to the finger.
2. The punch is rotated in 1 direction with continuous and mild pressure.
3. The tissue is then carefully extracted with the help of iris scissors, trying not to use forceps, to avoid crushing the specimen.
4. No suture is necessary.

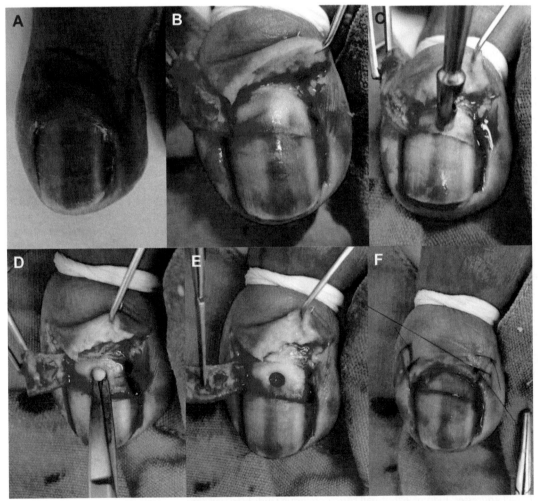

Fig. 1. Technique for medial melanonychia (*A*). Cutting and elevating proximal nail plate (*B*). Performing a 3-mm punch biopsy (*C*). Removal of tissue (*D*). Circular defect (*E*). Reattachment and suture of nail plate and fold (*F*).

If the nail plate is present, it has to be removed before biopsy. This is the best way it can be done:

1. The nail plate can be removed with a bigger punch (4 mm).
2. The nail plate is removed and the underlying nail bed is exposed.
3. A smaller punch (2–3 mm) is used to for a biopsy of the nail bed.
4. The nail plate is reinserted and may be fixed with cyanoacrylate glue or by suturing the nail plate to the nail fold (**Fig. 1**).[3]

Another way to remove the nail plate is to cut the desired shape of the nail plate with a scalpel. The submarine technique can also be used.[4] This technique consists of removing a strip of nail plate or total avulsion. The submarine technique is used when the site for the tissue sampling has been explored previously.

A punch biopsy can be used in every anatomic site of the nail apparatus (**Fig. 2**). It is helpful in diagnosing nail disorders, but can also be useful for treating subungual abscess or hematoma (**Fig. 3**). A modified nail punch biopsy technique consists in using a 2-mm punch for trepanation of the nail plate (**Table 1**).[5]

POTENTIAL COMPLICATIONS AND THEIR MANAGEMENT

Some complications can be expected, including edema and pain. These complications can be prevented by elevating the extremities. The hand may be elevated using a sling. Infection, although rare, is an unexpected complication that should be treated immediately after it is suspected with oral broad spectrum antibiotics.

POSTPROCEDURAL CARE

A thick dressing is secured and kept in place for 48 hours to prevent excessive bleeding and to protect the area from trauma and pain. The patient should be careful to rest for at least 1 week to avoid swelling, pain, and other potential complications. After 2 days the patient will need to clean the surgical site with peroxide on a daily basis and apply a petrolatum gauze to prevent objects from sticking to the wound.[2]

OUTCOMES

If any, permanent nail dystrophy or hemorrhage may occur.

EVIDENCE: CLINICAL RESULTS IN THE LITERATURE

A proximal nail fold–lunula double punch technique has been recently published and it seems to have

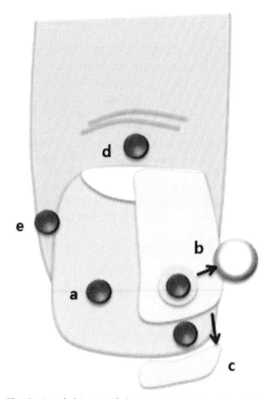

Fig. 2. Punch biopsy of the nail apparatus. Punch biopsy may be performed on the nail bed (a). On the nail bed when the nail plate is present, a bigger punch must first be used to expose the nail bed (b). On the nail bed with the submarine technique, which exposes the distal end of the nail bed by clipping the nail plate (c), on the proximal (d) or lateral nail fold (e).

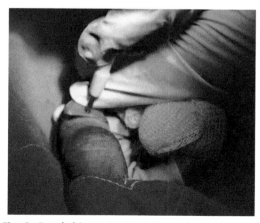

Fig. 3. Punch biopsy to treat a complete subungual hematoma. A punch is positioned perpendicular to the nail plate to evacuate a hematoma.

Table 1
Indications for punch biopsy according to anatomic site

| Anatomic Site | Uses | |
	Diagnosis	Treatment
Nail plate	Onicomicosis Hematomas	—

Periungual folds
  Hyponychium
  Eponychium
  Lateral folds
	Tumors
	Inflammatory conditions
		Tumors
		Warts

Matrix	Inflammatory conditions Longitudinal melanonychia Tumors	Tumors Longitudinal melanonychia
Nail bed	Inflammatory conditions Eritronychia	Subungual hematoma Acute paronychia

good results for tissue sampling. It avoids having to cut the proximal nail fold to expose the matrix. According to the authors, it is less painful, has faster cure rates, and fewer possibilities for dystrophy.[1]

SUMMARY

A punch biopsy can be used for the diagnosis and treatment of nail conditions in all areas of the nail apparatus. When the procedure is performed with a careful handling of the anatomic site and specimen, a successful diagnosis can be achieved in most cases.

SUPPLEMENTARY DATA

Supplementary data related to this article can be found online at http://dx.doi.org/10.1016/j.det.2014.12.008.

REFERENCES

1. Kim JE, Ahn HS, Cheon MS, et al. Proximal nail fold-lunula double punch technique: a less invasive method for sampling nail matrix without nail avulsion. Indian J Dermatol Venereol Leprol 2011; 77(3):346–8.
2. Haneke E. Nail surgery indications and outcomes. Expert Rev Dermatol 2006;1(1):1–11.
3. Domínguez Cherit J, Fonte Avalos V, Gutiérrez Mendoza D. Principios Básicos en cirugía de uñas. En UÑAS. Mexico City (México): Elsevier; 2011. p. 42–58.
4. Zaiac M, Norton ES, Tosti A. The "submarine hatch" nail bed biopsy. J Am Acad Dermatol 2014; 70:E128.
5. Khan A, Wes E, Tyler M. Two-millimeter biopsy punch. A painless instrument for evacuation of subungueal haematomas in adults and children. J Hand Surg Eur 2011;36:615.

Best Way to Treat an Ingrown Toenail

Nilton Di Chiacchio, MD, PhD[a],*, Nilton Gioia Di Chiacchio, MD[a,b]

KEYWORDS

- Ingrown toenail • Toe • Toenail procedures • Nail phenolization • Nail plate • Debulking
- Nail hypertrophy

KEY POINTS

- Nail phenolization is considered a useful procedure for treating ingrowing toenails.
- Nail phenolization is indicated when partial and definitive removal of the nail plate is necessary.
- Nail phenolization is simple and inexpensive, and associated with little postoperative discomfort, a quick return to normal activities, and a low rate of complication and recurrence.
- The Howard-Dubois and super U techniques are indicated when ingrowing nails are caused by hypertrophy of nail folds, according to the degree of severity.
- The Howard-Dubois and super U techniques produce very good results, although the healing time and time until return to normal activities are longer with the super U technique.

An ingrown toenail is a common problem that causes significant morbidity and disability in daily life. An imbalance between the widths of the nail plate and the nail bed and the hypertrophy of nail folds are considered to be the causes.[1] A large number of articles on the conservative treatment of ingrowing toenails have been described.[2–6] Techniques such as massaging the nail folds, taping, gutter splinting, and orthesis may help in the treatment of ingrowing nails, especially in mild cases and in children. These treatments are lengthy and, when they are not well indicated, recurrence rates are considered high.[7] Surgical treatment is indicated either when conservative treatments have failed or in moderate and severe cases.[1] For cases in which nail is responsible for the ingrown toenail, the definitive narrowing of the nail plate is preferred. When the condition is caused by hypertrophy of nail folds, debulking of the periungueal soft tissues is performed.[1] This article describes the best surgical treatment of ingrowing toenails.

NARROWING OF THE NAIL PLATE

Nail phenolization is the best technique for definitive narrowing of the nail plate.[7] It is well indicated in patients with diabetes and those using anticoagulants.[8] Patients should be advised about the postoperative oozing and inflammatory process of proximal and lateral nail folds, and normal daily activities.

Nail phenolization is considered easy to perform, but specialized training is required. After cleaning the involved digit with alcohol 70%, a tourniquet is applied and distal block anesthesia with lidocaine 2% without epinephrine is administered. When granulation tissue is present, it should be curetted to enable a better view of the nail plate to avoid excessive nail plate removal. The lateral involved nail plate is detached from the nail bed and the lateral and proximal nail folds ($\approx$3–5 mm). The nail plate is split using a scissors or nail nippers from the free edge to the matrix and removed using a hemostat in a rotation motion.

[a] Dermatologic Clinic, Hospital do Servidor Público Municipal de São Paulo, São Paulo, Brazil; [b] Department of Dermatology, Medical School of ABC, São Paulo, Brazil
* Corresponding author. Rua Machado Pedrosa, 370, Sao Paulo 02045010, Brazil.
E-mail address: ndichia@terra.com.br

Dermatol Clin 33 (2015) 277–282
http://dx.doi.org/10.1016/j.det.2014.12.009

When necessary, the nail matrix, nail bed, and lateral nail fold are gently curetted to remove debris. A cotton swab is moistened with phenol solution 88% and applied to the lateral sulcus under the proximal fold and rubbed vigorously onto the matrix for 1 minute (**Fig. 1**).[9]

Management of Complications

Oozing appears on the third day and may continue for up to 3 weeks. This oozing is improved by frequent washing of the wound, at least twice a day.[9] A 20% ferric chloride solution can be used just after phenolization to improve postoperative drainage.[10] Slight edema in the lateral and proximal nail folds may remain for 1 week, and can be improved by applying clobetasol cream. Infection, although rare, is the most common complication. An antibiotic is indicated in the case of postoperative infection.[11] Unnecessary burn of proximal and lateral nail folds appears when the cotton swab is excessively moistened; the applicator must be moistened with phenol solution, but not dripping.[9] Postoperative periostitis may occur when the nail matrix is strongly curetted. This procedure, when necessary, must be performed gently.[12] Excessive detachment of the nail plate plus a dripping applicator may result in a temporary or definitive nail dystrophy. Care must be given to detach just the necessary lateral part of the nail plate.[9]

Postprocedural Care

The limb should be elevated for 1 day. The dressing should be removed after 24 hours and the wound cleaned with 3% hydrogen peroxide. The patient should be advised to wash the wound twice a day and avoid closed shoes until the oozing disappears. The wound should be covered with a simple bandage. Patients should return for follow-up the next day and in 10, 30, and 60 days.

The clinical results and a review of the literature are summarized in **Table 1**.[13–16]

Outcomes

The results of nail phenolization are considered excellent, both functionally and cosmetically (**Fig. 2**).

DEBULKING OF THE PERIUNGUEAL SOFT TISSUE

When an ingrowing nail is caused by hypertrophy of the nail folds, 2 different surgeries can be performed. The Howard-Dubois procedure is the best technique for mild to moderate cases,[1] whereas the super U procedure is best for severe cases.[17]

Howard-Dubois Procedure

After cleaning the digit involved with alcohol 70%, a tourniquet is applied and distal block anesthesia

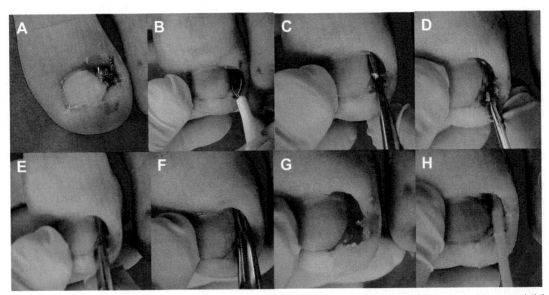

Fig. 1. Technique of nail matrix phenolization. (*A*) Lateral ingrown toenail. (*B*) Granulation tissue is curetted. (*C*) Nail plate is detached from the proximal nail fold. (*D*) Nail plate is detached from nail bed. (*E*) Nail plate is cut from the free edge to the mail matrix. (*F*) Nail plate is removed using rotation motion. (*G*) The wound is cleaned. (*H*) Phenol solution (88%) is applied on the nail matrix with a cotton swab.

Table 1			
Recurrence rates of nail matrix phenolization			
Author, Year	Number of Surgeries	Follow-up (mo)	Recurrence Rate (%)
Kimata et al,[13] 1995	537	6	1.1
Bostanci et al,[14] 2001	350	25	0.6
Andreassi et al,[15] 2004	948	18	4.3
Di Chiacchio et al,[16] 2010	267	33	1.9

Data from Refs.[13–16]

with lidocaine 2% without epinephrine is administered. A fish-mouth incision is made parallel to the distal groove around the tip of the toe, 5 mm below the distal and lateral grooves, running from the medial to the lateral aspect of the distal interphalangeal joint. A second incision is performed to create a wedge of approximately 7 mm at its greatest width in the middle of the distal wall. The crescent is removed using a sharp-pointed scissors. The wound edges must be approximated to determine whether enough tissue has been removed. If not, a new strip should be re-excised from the lower edge of the wound. Fat and fibrous tissue must be removed from the wound to ease the closure. The suture may be performed with simple interrupted stitches (nylon 4-0 or 5-0) or running lock stitches to avoid bleeding (**Fig. 3**).[17]

Management of complications
Complications are unusual. Necrosis is possible in cases of overtightened sutures.

Postprocedural care
A very greasy nonadherent dressing covered with dry cotton is used to avoid bleeding. The dressing is replaced after 24 hours. The limb should be elevated for 48 hours. Pain is minimal to moderate, and analgesics should be prescribed. Stitches are removed after 14 days.

Outcomes
The nail plate grows normally and the cosmetic results are excellent with the Howard-Dubois technique (**Fig. 4**).

Super U Procedure

This technique described by Rosa[18] is very well indicated in cases of severe hypertrophy of nail folds. Patients should be advised that daily activities will be compromised during the postoperative period because of the long healing time (up to 2 months).

After proximal or distal block anesthesia is administered, a tourniquet is applied and a U-shaped incision is performed from the proximal part of lateral nail fold, running through to the distal nail fold, and ending on the other side of lateral nail fold, comprising the whole hypertrophic tissue. A second incision begins on the lateral nail groove, in the same place as the first one, extending to the digit where the first incision ended. The hypertrophic tissue is held with a sturdy Adson forceps, and pulled to allow the tissue to be removed at bone contact with a sharp-pointed scissors. A running lock stitch, with nonabsorbable 3-0 or 4-0 suture, is performed around the first incision to avoid bleeding (**Fig. 5**).

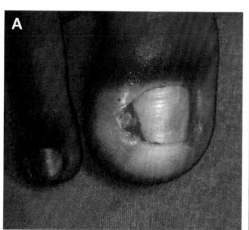
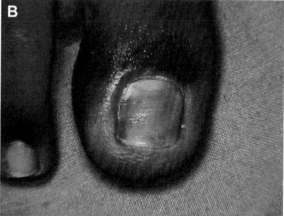

Fig. 2. (*A*) Ingrown toenail of the lateral side. (*B*) Outcome after 3 months.

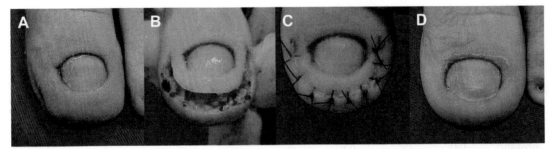

Fig. 3. Howard-Dubois technique. (*A*) A moderate case of ingrown toenail (lateral and distal). (*B*) Removal of skin and fat from one side to the other of the distal interphalangeal joint. (*C*) Suture with nylon 4-0. (*D*) Outcome after 2 months.

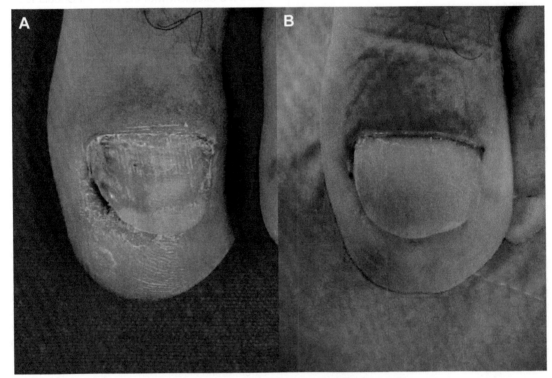

Fig. 4. Howard-Dubois technique. (*A*) Before surgery. (*B*) Outcome after 2 months.

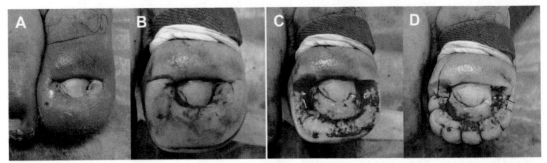

Fig. 5. Super U technique. (*A*) Severe ingrown toenail (lateral and distal) with lateral granulation tissue. (*B*) Transverse incision from the proximal nail fold, running parallel with lateral and distal edge of the nail, from one side to the other. (*C*) Hypertrophic tissue is removed. (*D*) Running lock suture with nonabsorbable 4-0 suture.

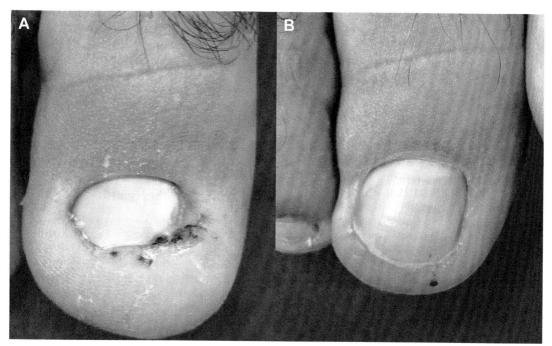

Fig. 6. (*A*) Severe ingrown toenail with hypertrophy of lateral and distal nail folds. (*B*) Outcome 6 months after super U technique.

Postprocedural care

Alginate dressing is useful to cover the wound. A secondary dressing with dry cotton, covered with layers of mesh gauze, is applied on the alginate. All of the dressing is covered with a narrow elastic bandage, allowing precise pressure over the wound. The limb must be elevated for 2 days and painkillers are prescribed. The dressing is removed after 2 days by the surgeon. The wound is washed with 3% hydrogen peroxide solution to remove the remaining blood, and saline solution 0.9% and a simple dressing with a greasy antiseptic ointment is applied and renewed twice daily until healing is complete. Closed shoes should be avoided during the healing time.

Management of potential complications

Severe pain during the first 48 hours is common. Mild opioid-type narcotic analgesics (eg, dextropropoxyphene, tramadol, naloxone associated with tilidine) should be prescribed.

Infection is rare if the wound is cleaned twice daily. In cases of infection, antibiotics should be prescribed.

Outcomes

Despite the long healing time, the improvement is dramatic with the super U technique (**Fig. 6**).

SUMMARY

Nail phenolization is considered a useful procedure for treating ingrowing toenails. It is indicated when partial and definitive removal of the nail plate is necessary. It is simple and inexpensive, and associated with little postoperative discomfort, a quick return to normal activities, and a low rate of complication and recurrence. The results are cosmetically acceptable.

The Howard-Dubois and super U techniques are indicated when ingrowing nails are caused by hypertrophy of nail folds, according to the degree of severity. Both techniques produce very good results, although the healing time and time until return to normal activities are longer with the super U technique.

REFERENCES

1. Richert B. Surgical management of ingrown toenails - an update overdue. Dermatol Ther 2012;25(6): 498–509.

2. Arai H, Arai T, Nakajima H, et al. Simple and effective treatment for ingrowing nail. Rinsho Derma (Tokyo) 2002;44:1321–8.

3. Arai H, Arai T, Haneke E. Simple and effective conservative treatment for ingrowing nails (Acrylic affixed gutter splint, sculptured nail and anchor

taping methods). Rinsho Derma (Tokyo) 2010; 52(11):1604–13.

4. Arai H, Arai T, Haneke E. Simple and effective non-invasive treatment methods for ingrown and pincer nail including acrylic affixed gutter splint, anchor taping, sculptures nails, shape memory alloy nail clip and plastic nail braces as well as 40% urea past. J Kochi Med Ass 2011; 16:37–56.

5. Arai H, Arai T, Haneke E. Treatment of ingrown and pincer nail using acrylic affixed gutter splint, anchor taping and a shape memory alloy nail clip (Cu-AlMn). MB Derma 2011;184:108–19.

6. Di Chiacchio N, Kadunc BV, Trindade de Almeida AR, et al. Treatment of transverse overcurvature of the nail with a plastic device: measurement of response. J Am Acad Dermatol 2006;55(6):1081–4.

7. Eekhof JA, Van Wijk B, Knuistingh Neven A, et al. Interventions for ingrowing toenails. Cochrane Database Syst Rev 2012;(4):CD001541.

8. Felton PM, Weaver TD. Phenol and alcohol chemical matrixectomy in diabetic versus nondiabetic patients. A retrospective study. J Am Podiatr Med Assoc 1999;89(8):410–2.

9. Di Chiacchio N, Richert B, Haneke E. Surgery of the matrix. In: Richert B, Di Chiacchio N, Haneke E, editors. Nail surgery. 1st edition. London: Healthcare; 2010. p. 106.

10. Aksakal AB, Atahan C, Oztaş P, et al. Minimizing postoperative drainage with 20% ferric chloride after chemical matricectomy with phenol. Dermatol Surg 2001;27(2):158–60.

11. Dovison R, Keenan AM. Wound healing and infection in nail matrix phenolization wounds. Does topical medication make a difference? J Am Podiatr Med Assoc 2001;91(5):230–3.

12. Tassara G, Machado MA, Gouthier MA. Treatment of ingrown nail: comparison of recurrence rates between the nail matrix phenolization classical technique and phenolization associated with nail matrix curettage - is the association necessary? An Bras Dermatol 2011;86(5):1046–8.

13. Kimata Y, Uetake M, Tsukada S, et al. Follow-up study of patients treated for ingrown nails with the nail matrix phenolization method. Plast Reconstr Surg 1995;95(4):719–24.

14. Bostanci S, Ekmekçi P, Gürgey E. Chemical matricectomy with phenol for the treatment of ingrowing toenail: a review of the literature and follow-up of 172 treated patients. Acta Derm Venereol 2001; 81(3):181–3.

15. Andreassi A, Grimaldi L, D'Aniello C, et al. Segmental phenolization for the treatment of ingrowing toenails: a review of 6 years experience. J Dermatolog Treat 2004;15(3):179–81.

16. Di Chiacchio N, Belda W Jr, Di Chiacchio NG, et al. Nail matrix phenolization for treatment of ingrowing nail: technique report and recurrence rate of 267 surgeries. Dermatol Surg 2010;36(4):534–7.

17. Richert B. Surgery of the lateral nail folds. In: Richert B, Di Chiacchio N, Haneke E, editors. Nail surgery. 1st edition. London: Healthcare; 2010. p. 89.

18. Rosa IP. Hipercurvatura transversa da lamina ungueal e lamina ungueal que não cresce. Remoção do "U" largo de pele, osteocorreção do leito e cicatrização por segunda intenção (Tese). São Paulo (Brazil): Universidade Federal de São Paulo, Escola Paulista de Medicina; 2005. p. 156.

Best Way to Remove a Subungual Tumor

Jonathan Weiss, MD[a], Martin N. Zaiac, MD[b,c],*

KEYWORDS

• Nail surgery • Subungual tumor • Surgical techniques • Surgical pearls

KEY POINTS

• The techniques for basic removal of subungual tumors can be mastered by dermatologists with a good understanding of the anatomy of the nail unit.
• It is important to keep in mind the goal of the procedure and the desired outcome given the clinical context of the subungual tumor.
• A good medical history should be obtained to assess for factors that can increase the risk of complications, and a thorough examination including imaging is usually indicated to evaluate the extent the tumor.
• Complete nail plate avulsion is rarely indicated for the removal of subungual tumors, and numerous less morbid partial avulsion techniques have been described in the literature.
• The more common adverse outcomes are generally mild and well accepted by the patient, while serious complications are rare.

 A video of a submarine hatch nail biopsy accompanies this article at http://www.derm.theclinics.com/

INTRODUCTION

Subungual tumors encompass a multitude of benign and malignant entities that originate from the nail matrix or the nail bed. Although these tumors are relatively uncommon in the general population, they are often brought to the attention of a dermatologist for diagnosis and treatment. These patients usually present due to dissatisfaction with the appearance of a visible nail abnormality or due to symptoms such as pain, tenderness, or discomfort.[1] Many dermatologists, however, are not comfortable with diagnosing and/or treating such patients due to lack of training. A survey of third-year dermatology residents demonstrated that only 10% had performed more than 10 nail procedures, and up to 30% had not performed any at all.[2] Nevertheless, the techniques for performing nail surgery are not too different from standard dermatologic surgery. With a good understanding of the unique anatomy of the nail unit and enough experience, nail surgery techniques can be mastered, and these procedures can be performed comfortably and safely in an outpatient dermatology clinic.

TREATMENT GOALS AND PLANNED OUTCOMES

When planning a surgical procedure to remove a subungual tumor, it is imperative to keep in mind the goal of the procedure and the desired

Disclosures: No relevant conflicts of interest to disclose.
[a] Department of Dermatology & Cutaneous Surgery, University of Miami Miller School of Medicine, 1600 Northwest 10th Avenue, RMSB 2023A, Miami, FL 33136, USA; [b] Department of Dermatology, Herbert Wertheim College of Medicine, Florida International University, 11200 SW 8th Street, AHC2, Miami, FL 33199, USA; [c] Greater Miami Skin and Laser Center, Mount Sinai Medical Center, 4308 Alton Road, Suite 750, Miami Beach, FL 33140, USA
* Corresponding author. Greater Miami Skin and Laser Center, Mount Sinai Medical Center, 4308 Alton Road, Suite 750, Miami Beach, FL 33140.
E-mail address: drmartyz@aol.com

Dermatol Clin 33 (2015) 283–287
http://dx.doi.org/10.1016/j.det.2014.12.010
0733-8635/15/$ – see front matter © 2015 Elsevier Inc. All rights reserved

outcome. One must consider individual factors for each case in order to decide on the appropriate technique. Although some subungual tumors have pathognomonic clinical features or characteristic symptomatology, a definitive diagnosis can sometimes only be rendered with adequate histopathological evaluation. In many instances, particularly when differentiating between benign and malignant entities, an accurate diagnosis will greatly alter the patient's prognosis and subsequent management. In these cases, the goal of the procedure will be to sample the entire tumor or at least a substantial representative portion in order to obtain a definitive diagnosis. When a benign subungual tumor can be diagnosed clinically with relative certainty, as in the case of a glomus tumor or an onychomatricoma, then the removal of this tumor can be planned with the aim of restoring functionality, mitigating unacceptable symptoms, or achieving improved cosmesis. Lastly, complete removal with clear margins should be the goal when a malignant diagnosis of a subungual tumor has been confirmed, and the appropriate techniques should be utilized to maximize the chance for cure and minimize the rate of recurrence.

PREOPERATIVE PLANNING AND PREPARATION

In planning the procedure, a proper medical history should be obtained in order to assess for possible risk factors that can increase chances of complications. Some of these risk factors include a history of smoking, diabetes, peripheral vascular disease, Raynaud phenomenon, immunocompromised states, and the use of antiplatelet or anticoagulation therapy. Imaging of the affected digit should be obtained to evaluate the extent or localization of the tumor. Plain film radiography can be helpful in evaluating tumor involvement or invasion into the bone, while MRI can also help identify the exact location of a tumor and its relationship to surrounding structures.[3] In the case of malignant tumors, clinical examination of regional lymph nodes should be completed, as the presence of lymphadenopathy should trigger further work-up for lymphatic spread of the tumor.

Prior to the procedure, the affected extremity should be examined for any signs of infection or compromised perfusion. The patient should also be assessed to determine if prophylactic antibiotics are warranted.[4] The goals of the planned procedure and expected outcomes should be discussed with the patient; additionally, the risks and benefits should be explained in detail, and a signed written consent form should be obtained.

PATIENT POSITIONING

Patients should be sitting or lying comfortably. The particular extremity should be positioned in a comfortable and neutral position, while allowing the hand or foot to be placed flat on a firm surface with the dorsal aspect exposed. It is important to ensure that the positioning is also comfortable for the surgeon.

BEST WAY TO REMOVE A SUBUNGUAL TUMOR

There are many approaches to removing a subungual tumor; however, all methods share in common some basic, yet crucial preparatory steps. An essential requirement of any nail procedure is to ensure adequate anesthesia given the highly sensitive area. Anesthetic techniques for nail procedures are discussed in detail separately in this publication. It is advised that the patient copiously scrub the affected hand or foot with soap and warm water prior to the procedure in order to remove potential contaminants. The area is then prepared and draped in sterile fashion. Generally, chlorhexidine is preferred as a surgical preparation over providone–iodine solution.[5,6] For procedures on the hand, a sterile glove can be worn by the patient with a small hole cut on the distal end of the corresponding finger. This technique further establishes a sterile surgical field, and provides an effective tourniquet if the glove finger is rolled back to snuggly fit on the proximal portion of the finger.[5–8] When surgery is performed on the toenails, a sterile penrose drain can be used as a tourniquet to obtain a bloodless field. Although not widely used, commercially available T-ring digital tourniquets are relatively inexpensive and have been shown to provide reliable hemostasis at lower overall pressures than other techniques.[9,10] Regardless of the chosen method, it is crucial to release the tourniquet every 20 to 30 minutes to avoid tissue ischemia caused by prolonged hypoxia. The use of sterile versus nonsterile gloves for the surgeon and assistants is a debated issue in dermatologic surgery, with a recent study demonstrating no difference in rate of infection for resection and reconstruction in Mohs micrographic surgery.[11]

Variations in the surgical techniques for removal of a subungual tumor arise from different methods to complete two main steps of the procedure: (1) visualizing or accessing the tumor in the nail bed or nail matrix and (2) extirpating the tumor itself. Although preference and experience of the surgeon play important roles, tumor location and the objective of the procedure are the main determining factors in choosing a technique.

Classically, complete avulsion of the entire nail plate was preferred, as it allows for the best visualization of a subungual tumor. However, newer teaching supports the use of more elegant and less invasive methods whenever possible. Techniques that maximize the preservation of important attachments of the nail plate will facilitate the replacement of the nail plate after surgery. The replaced nail plate serves as a protective biologic dressing, expediting healing and decreasing postoperative morbidity.[12] The trap door avulsion is a commonly utilized technique that allows for extensive visualization of the hyponychium, nail bed, and distal nail matrix while still maintaining proximal attachment of the nail plate. This article will focus on the steps of the trap door avulsion as it is the workhorse of nail surgery, and most other partial avulsion techniques are variations from this method.

Once anesthesia is achieved, a nail elevator is first introduced underneath the distal free edge of the nail plate. While applying firm upward pressure, the elevator is advanced, separating the hyponychium. The elevator can then be carefully pushed forward while taking care to minimize injury to the underlying epithelium of the nail bed and nail matrix (**Fig. 1**). Once the nail plate has been entirely separated from the nail bed and distal nail matrix, the lateral attachments can be freed, and the nail plate can be reflected upwards with a hemostat or a suture (**Fig. 2**). The intact attachment to the proximal nail fold will give the nail plate the appearance of a trap door as suggested by the technique's name. Oblique skin incisions on both sides of the proximal nail fold can be employed to maximize the reflection of the nail plate and obtain more proximal exposure of the nail matrix.

Various other limited avulsion techniques with more focused reflection of the nail plate have been detailed in the literature, including the lateral and longitudinal partial nail plate avulsions,

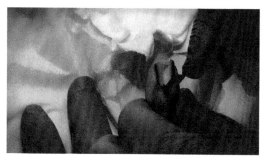

Fig. 2. After complete separation from the nail bed and nail matrix, the lateral attachments can be freed and the nail plate can be reflected upwards.

window nail plate avulsion, lateral nail plate curl, partial proximal nail plate avulsion,[12] and the submarine hatch (Video 1).[13]

After the desired exposure is obtained, the subungual tumor can be removed. When the margins of the tumor are not obvious, a diagnosis is not yet known, or complete removal is indicated, a longitudinal excision extending from the nail matrix to the distal nail bed is preferred. A number 15 blade is used to make longitudinal incisions down to the periosteum along both sides of the tumor with necessary margins, and sharp curved iris scissors can be used to excise the tissue (**Fig. 3**). Meticulous handling of the specimen will minimize trauma to this delicate tissue and maximize the value of histopathological examination. When exploration reveals a localized well-circumscribed tumor, as in the case of a subungual glomus tumor, removal with a punch tool can be an effective and less morbid alternative.[13,14] When an excisional biopsy of a broad lesion on the matrix is required for evaluation of longitudinal melanonychia, a tangential shave excision can adequately sample the entire lesion while minimizing subsequent nail plate dystrophy.[15–17] The details pertaining to the evaluation of longitudinal melanonychia are

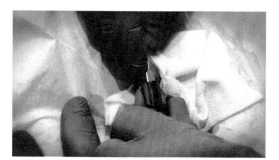

Fig. 1. A nail elevator is used to carefully separate the nail plate from the hyponychium, nail bed, and nail matrix.

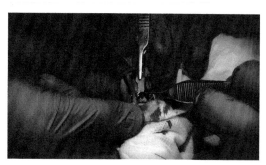

Fig. 3. A number 15 blade is used to make longitudinal incisions down to the periosteum along both sides of the tumor with necessary margins and the tumor is carefully excised.

discussed elsewhere in this publication. Mohs micrographic surgery is also a crucial technique in nail surgery. It is highly effective and ideal for margin control and the tissue-sparing removal of subungual nonmelanoma malignant tumors given the sensitive anatomy of the nail unit.[18–20]

POTENTIAL COMPLICATIONS AND MANAGEMENT OF THEM

Surgery of the nail unit is generally well tolerated by patients, and serious complications are rare.[9] The most common adverse outcomes include dystrophy of the nail plate caused by scarring of the nail matrix and onycholysis caused by scarring of the nail bed. This can be minimized if the breadth of the surgical defect spans no more than 3 mm. If the defect extends beyond this cutoff, careful approximation with sutures is warranted. Scarring of the proximal nail fold may result in a dorsal pterygium. Infections are uncommon and can be minimized by meticulous preoperative cleansing and sterilization. Postoperative oral antibiotics for prevention of surgical site infection are usually not indicated, but may be beneficial in certain high-risk individuals. Subungual hematomas are relatively uncommon, and may require drainage in some instances. Ischemia and tissue necrosis can be avoided by maintaining the tourniquet time under 20 to 30 minutes, and a good preoperative evaluation to assess for poor perfusion of the digit. Patients must be informed that a significant portion may develop some degree of dysesthesia; however, most patients experience resolution.[21]

POSTPROCEDURAL CARE

Following the procedure, the surgical site should be cleansed with normal saline and covered with a nonstick dressing such as petrolatum-impregnated gauze. A loose and well-padded bandage should then be secured with vertically oriented tape to avoid strangulation of the digit. The patient should be observed for at least 15 minutes to ensure there is no excessive bleeding and to avoid a vasovagal reaction. Whenever possible, the affected extremity should be elevated above the level of the heart to minimize bleeding and decrease edema by improving venous return. The bandage should remain in place for 24 hours, and then changed once to twice a day with adequate cleansing using soap and water prior to applying a new dressing. Analgesia with acetaminophen is preferred over nonsteroidal anti-inflammatory medications, as it does not affect platelet function. Occasionally, opiates are necessary for short-term control of postprocedural pain. The authors generally have their patients follow-up in 1 week, or sooner as needed if any complications arise.

SUMMARY

Subungual tumors are uncommon, but they are encountered by dermatologists with relative frequency. Dermatologists should not be discouraged in these cases. Simple surgical techniques such as those described in this publication can be followed to safely and effectively remove subungual tumors in the clinic.

SUPPLEMENTARY DATA

Supplementary data related to this article can be found online at http://dx.doi.org/10.1016/j.det. 2014.12.010.

REFERENCES

1. de Berker DA, Dahl MG, Comaish JS, et al. Nail surgery: an assessment of indications and outcome. Acta Derm Venereol 1996;76(6):484–7.
2. Lee EH, Nehal KS, Dusza SW, et al. Procedural dermatology training during dermatology residency: a survey of third-year dermatology residents. J Am Acad Dermatol 2011;64(3):475–83.
3. Goettmann S, Drape JL, Idy-Peretti I, et al. Magnetic resonance imaging: a new tool in the diagnosis of tumours of the nail apparatus. Br J Dermatol 1994; 130(6):701–10.
4. Wright TI, Baddour LM, Berbari EF, et al. Antibiotic prophylaxis in dermatologic surgery: advisory statement 2008. J Am Acad Dermatol 2008;59(3):464–73.
5. Jellinek NJ. Nail surgery: practical tips and treatment options. Dermatol Ther 2007;20(1):68–74.
6. Haneke E. Nail surgery. Clin Dermatol 2013;31(5): 516–25.
7. Harrington AC, Cheyney JM, Kinsley-Scott T, et al. A novel digital tourniquet using a sterile glove and hemostat. Dermatol Surg 2004;30:1065–7.
8. McGinness LJ, Parlette HL 3rd. Versatile sterile field for nail surgery using a sterile glove. Dermatol Online J 2005;11(3):10.
9. Findley A, Lee K, Jellinek NJ. Nail surgery among Mohs surgeons: prevalence, safety, and practice patterns. Dermatol Surg 2014;40(6):691–5.
10. Lahham S, Tu K, Ni M, et al. Comparison of pressures applied by digital tourniquets in the emergency department. West J Emerg Med 2011;12(2): 242–9.
11. Mehta D, Chambers N, Adams B, et al. Comparison of the prevalence of surgical site infection with use of sterile versus nonsterile gloves for resection and reconstruction during Mohs surgery. Dermatol Surg 2014;40(3):234–9.

12. Collins SC, Cordova K, Jellinek NJ. Alternatives to complete nail plate avulsion. J Am Acad Dermatol 2008;59(4):619–26.

13. Zaiac MN, Norton ES, Tosti A. The "submarine hatch" nail bed biopsy. J Am Acad Dermatol 2014; 70(6):e127–8.

14. Micheletti R, Sobanko J, Rubin A. Distal matrix glomus tumor presenting as longitudinal erythronychia: a pearl for surgical management. Dermatol Surg 2012;38(1):133–4.

15. Haneke E, Baran R. Longitudinal melanonychia. Dermatol Surg 2001;27(6):580–4.

16. Richert B, Theunis A, Norrenberg S, et al. Tangential excision of pigmented nail matrix lesions responsible for longitudinal melanonychia: evaluation of the technique on a series of 30 patients. J Am Acad Dermatol 2013;69(1):96–104.

17. Di Chiacchio N, Loureiro WR, Michalany NS, et al. Tangential biopsy thickness versus lesion depth in longitudinal melanonychia: a pilot study. Dermatol Res Pract 2012;2012:353864.

18. Zaiac MN, Weiss E. Mohs micrographic surgery of the nail unit and squamous cell carcinoma. Dermatol Surg 2001;27(3):246–51.

19. Goldminz D, Bennett RG. Mohs micrographic surgery of the nail unit. J Dermatol Surg Oncol 1992; 18(8):721–6.

20. Dika E, Piraccini BM, Balestri R, et al. Mohs surgery for squamous cell carcinoma of the nail: report of 15 cases. Our experience and a long-term follow up. Br J Dermatol 2012;167(6):1310–4.

21. Walsh ML, Shipley DV, de Berker DA. Survey of patients' experiences after nail surgery. Clin Exp Dermatol 2009;34(5):e154–6.

Diagnostic Applications of Nail Clippings

Sasha Stephen, MD[a], Antonella Tosti, MD[d],*, Adam I. Rubin, MD[a,b,c]

KEYWORDS

- Nail clipping • Nail pathology • Onychomycosis • Melanonychia • Onychomatricoma
- Subungual hematoma • Nail psoriasis • Nail cosmetics

KEY POINTS

- There is substantial overlap in the histologic features of nail unit psoriasis and onychomycosis in a nail clipping specimen, therefore a fungal stain is essential to diagnose onychomycosis.
- Use of nail softening agents in the preparation of nail clippings can substantially improve the tissue quality and histologic evaluation.
- Diaminobenzidine staining is useful in confirming the presence of hemorrhage in a nail clipping specimen.
- Fontana staining of a nail clipping can be helpful in localizing the origin of pigmentation within the nail matrix in cases of melanonychia.
- Nail clipping specimens can be used for perpetrator DNA and heavy metal poisoning evaluation in forensics.

INTRODUCTION

Nail clipping is one of the simplest diagnostic techniques performed in medicine, but it is often underused in the diagnosis of disease. Compared with many other tests in medicine, both patients and physicians have an instant familiarity with the procedure, because nail clippings are performed as part of routine grooming procedures. The benefits of performing nail clipping for diagnostic purposes are numerous, including minimal risk to the patient, increased diagnostic information about a nail disorder, rapid completion in the office, and in some cases the preparation of permanent glass slides that can be referred to in the future for further diagnostic study.

Dermatoses affecting the nail unit can be difficult to diagnose. Infectious, inflammatory, and neoplastic disorders of the nail unit can mimic each other on clinical examination.[1] Histopathology is helpful, and often necessary, to establish a specific diagnosis and to distinguish such similar-appearing entities. However, the need for tissue diagnosis can lead to unease, because clinicians are often reluctant to obtain a soft tissue biopsy specimen from the nail unit. Barriers to obtaining a soft tissue specimen from the nail unit include concern for a subsequent permanent nail unit dystrophy, lack of prior training in nail unit surgery, and the perceived technical difficulty of a nail unit biopsy.[2]

As opposed to obtaining a soft tissue specimen from the nail unit, obtaining a nail clipping does not require any specialized training, and can be used to evaluate a wide range of nail disorders. This article describes a variety of uses of nail clippings to help diagnose dermatoses of the nail unit, as well as best practices in order to obtain the

Conflicts of interest: None.
[a] Department of Dermatology, Hospital of the University of Pennsylvania, 3600 Spruce Street, 2 Maloney, Philadelphia, PA 19104, USA; [b] The Children's Hospital of Philadelphia, Philadelphia, PA 19104, USA; [c] Perelman School of Medicine at the University of Pennsylvania, Philadelphia, PA 19104, USA; [d] Department of Dermatology and Cutaneous Surgery, Miller School of Medicine, University of Miami, 1600 Northwest 10th Avenue, RMSB 2023A, Locator Code R-250 Miami, FL 33136, USA
* Corresponding author.
E-mail address: Atosti@med.miami.edu

Dermatol Clin 33 (2015) 289–301
http://dx.doi.org/10.1016/j.det.2014.12.011
0733-8635/15/$ – see front matter © 2015 Elsevier Inc. All rights reserved.

specimen, and correlate the findings within the specific clinical context. This article covers the use of nail clippings for the diagnosis of onychomycosis, nail unit psoriasis, subungual hematoma, and onychomatricoma (OM), and for forensics, surgical planning for nail unit biopsy of melanonychia, as well as distinguishing nail cosmetics from other dermatoses.

BEST PRACTICES FOR OBTAINING A NAIL CLIPPING FOR HISTOPATHOLOGIC EXAMINATION

In order to maximize diagnostic yield from a nail clipping, it is important to obtain a sample that is at least 4 mm in length. A common error is collecting a sample that is too small. If a very small sample is submitted, the nail plate tissue that is examined may not be representative of the overall pathologic process in the nail unit. In addition, a tiny sample may be damaged during routine laboratory processing procedures, and not survive the process. If a patient's nail is not long enough to obtain a sufficient sample, the patient should allow the nail to grow, and return to have a nail clipping at a later date. It may be useful to have the office staff explain to patients who are being evaluated for a nail problem, either verbally or in preprepared paperwork that is mailed to patients before their visits, that they should allow their nails to grow to a sufficient length and, in particular, should not clip their own nails before evaluation.

If the clinician is interested in performing a fungal culture in addition to the nail clipping, the target nail should be cleansed either with an alcohol swab or soap and water before clipping the nail, but this step is not required for histologic assessment alone. Cleansing the nail helps to remove the presence of any contaminating bacteria. There are a variety of nail instruments that can be used to obtain the nail clipping. A dual-action nail nipper is particularly helpful because of its hinged shape, and can create a large force at the point of clipping, making the clipping easier, especially of thick nails (**Fig. 1A**). A heavy-duty nail nipper may be used as well. Routine nail clippers, as are used by laypersons at home, are not recommended to obtain nail clippings in the medical office setting because of their inferiority compared with the aforementioned instruments.

When performing the nail clipping, the nail should be clipped as far back as possible without causing pain or bleeding. This method ensures that a sufficient sample is obtained and, in the case of onychomycosis, that the active area of infection is included. In the case of onychomycosis, if only a small distal sample of the nail plate is obtained, it may provide a false-negative result because of a sampling error. If onycholysis is present, the nail should be clipped back to the most proximal attachment of the nail plate to the nail bed. It is helpful to pathologists evaluating specimens to be provided with sufficient clinical context, as well as any special requests for

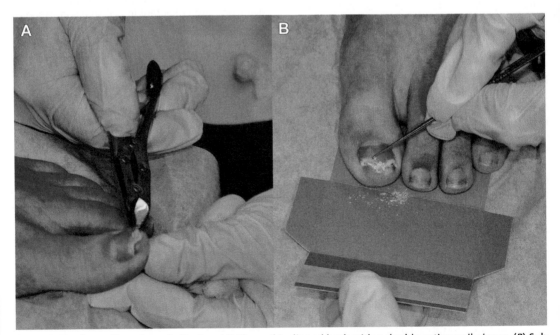

Fig. 1. Optimal sampling of a nail clipping. (*A*) The nail is clipped back with a double-action nail nipper. (*B*) Subungual debris is removed with a small curette and placed on a Dermapack.

processing or interpretation of the nail clipping specimen.

After the nail is clipped, and if a fungal culture is desired, a small curette can be used to gently dislodge any subungual material from the nail bed, which is sent for culture (see **Fig.** 1B). The clipped nail plate can be put into a formalin-filled bottle and sent to the pathology laboratory.

BEST PRACTICES FOR PREPARING A NAIL CLIPPING FOR HISTOPATHOLOGIC EXAMINATION

Because of the unique anatomy and physical characteristics of the nail unit, the pathology processing techniques required for nail clipping specimens are more complex than those for routine cutaneous specimens. The nail plate is rigid and often requires adequate softening to create high-quality sections, which in turn allow accurate diagnoses. There are numerous options for softening nail plate specimens, including 4% phenol, 5% trichloroacetic acid in 10% formalin, chitin-softening agent,[3] cedar oil, and 10% Tween 40, as well as sodium hydroxide (NaOH). André and colleagues[4] use Mollifex Gurr, dipping the paraffin blocks in it for 2 to 12 hours, depending on nail plate thickness.

A study by Lewin and colleagues[5] compared different methods of softening nail specimens for histologic sectioning. For nails of normal thickness, several methods were equally effective; namely, soaking in potassium hydroxide (KOH) or nitric acid after fixation in formaldehyde solution, or Tween 40 treatment of normally processed paraffin blocks. For thick nails, treatment with Tween 40 was preferred, although KOH was adequate.

Orchard and colleagues[6] performed an evaluation of several methods using softening agents to facilitate the preparation of reproducible, high-quality, formalin-fixed, paraffin-embedded sections of nail tissue. They collected nail plate specimens from 3 normal volunteers. The clippings were fixed in 10% neutral buffered formalin for 12 hours. Next the investigators applied the softening agents, including Veet (Reckitt Benckiser), Easy fabric conditioner (powder and liquid products), Fairy Liquid (Procter and Gamble), 30% KOH, and distilled water for 10 minutes each following paraffin wax embedding. The sections were cut at a thickness of 4 μm. The block was then faced off and treated with a different softener for evaluation. The investigators then evaluated sections taken after each softener was used and assessed the quality and number of sections before specimen damage became apparent. The

investigators found that Veet and Easy fabric conditioner were the best softening agents, closely followed by Fairy Liquid. These agents were superior to distilled water and 30% KOH, which provided fewer high-quality sections after application for 10 minutes.

Nazarian and colleagues[7] detailed a protocol using pretreatment with NaOH in the evaluation of 45 samples from fingernails and toenails of patients with clinically suspected onychomycosis. The specimens were soaked in 20% NaOH for 2 to 3 hours, then rinsed for 5 minutes under tap water before routine processing, paraffin embedding, and routine hematoxylin-eosin (H&E) periodic acid-Schiff (PAS) staining. This softening method provided higher-quality sections compared with no softening treatment. However, this study did not compare the quality of the specimens with that obtained using other softening agents. In addition, the investigators noted that NaOH treatment led to some areas of the nail plate having fainter PAS staining of fungal elements. However, this did not result in a false-negative diagnosis in any case. The investigators also suggested that NaOH may damage melanin and hemosiderin pigments, and therefore caution should be used when evaluating cases with clinical history of melanonychia.

Chang and colleagues[8] advocate using plastic embedding of nail plate specimens in 2-hydroxyethyl methacrylate as an alternative to softening agents, which allows thinner, uniform sections that adhere well to glass slides, and decreases the chance of dislodging the nail plate from the embedding media. However, the investigators note that this technique is technically difficult, costly, time consuming, and requires a motorized microtome and glass knives.

In our laboratory, we use 10% NaOH for pretreatment of nail plates. After a nail plate specimen is received in 10% formalin, the formalin is removed and replaced with 10% NaOH. The time of incubation is based on the size of the specimen. The specimens are monitored closely throughout the timing process to prevent degradation. Small specimens are incubated for approximately 45 minutes, whereas bigger specimens may be incubated for 2 to 3 hours. Once softening is completed, the nail plates are washed in running water for 10 minutes then returned for processing and embedding.

In order to help the nail specimens adhere to the glass slides, we coat the slides with a light film of adhesive solution and then let dry. This technique allows the nail to remain attached to the glass slides through H&E, special stain, and rigorous immunoperoxidase staining processes, if needed.

Otherwise, the tissue may fall off the slide and be lost. Once the tissue block is prepared, it is faced off and then allowed to sit in a tray containing 4% ammonium hydroxide for about 30 to 45 minutes before cutting to ensure easy passage of the knife through the nail clipping specimen. This step further ensures that the clippings adhere to the slide, because the adhesive solution alone may not suffice. Once the nail clipping sections are on the slide, the slides are placed in a 60° to 65°C oven for approximately 1 hour to allow the sections to dry sufficiently before proceeding with staining.

When assessing a nail clipping for onychomycosis in particular, it is important to keep in mind that hyphae, when present, are most commonly localized in areas of subungual hyperkeratosis and the ventral aspect of the nail plate. Given this phenomenon, Chang and colleagues[8] described a novel method of isolating subungual hyperkeratosis from the nail plate for histologic evaluation during the grossing stage of specimen preparation, before PAS staining for onychomycosis. After nail clippings were submitted to the laboratory, the subungual hyperkeratosis was trimmed from the base of the nail plate using standard grossing instruments. This subungual material was then processed directly without the need for additional steps of softening. The investigators report that this technique provided the diagnosis, such that fungal elements were identified in the samples, in 64 of 66 (97%) cases of onychomycosis. This method spared the added technical difficulty and cost of nail plate softening and processing. In 3% of the specimens in which the subungual hyperkeratosis was PAS negative, the nail plate was positive. Therefore, the investigators recommend that, in cases in which the PAS stain of the subungual debris is negative, sections of the nail plate should be examined to avoid false-negative results when using this technique.

Recently, there has been some debate regarding the fungal stain of choice for identifying hyphae for the diagnosis of onychomycosis. One study by D'Hue and colleagues[9] showed the superiority of Gomori methenamine silver (GMS) compared with PAS in detecting the presence of hyphae in nail plate biopsies. The investigators performed GMS staining on 20 PAS-positive and 51 PAS-negative nail clippings with a clinical diagnosis of onychomycosis. All 20 of the PAS-positive cases were GMS positive, and 5 of the PAS-negative cases were GMS positive. In addition, GMS stains were easier and less time consuming to interpret compared with PAS.

A similar study was performed by Reza Kermanshahi and Rhatigan.[10] These investigators compared PAS and GMS stains on sections from 30 cases of clinically suspected onychomycosis using sections cut at similar depths of the tissue blocks. The PAS stain was positive in 22 of 30 specimens, and GMS was positive in 19 of 30. On samples that were originally negative with GMS but positive with PAS, cutting deeper into the block revealed GMS positivity. The investigators therefore suggested that the two stains are equivalent for detecting the presence of hyphae. They also explain that although the PAS stain is simple to perform, the GMS stain can be technically difficult and requires experienced histotechnologists.[10]

A study of efficacy of histopathologic PAS staining of nail clippings by Mayer and colleagues[11] revealed that parakeratosis and globules of plasma were statistically significantly more common in the nail samples with fungal elements than in those without on examination of H&E-stained specimens. The investigators concluded that this finding may indicate an ongoing inflammatory process associated with onychomycosis.

Another study, by Barak and colleagues,[12] concluded that there was no difference in the sensitivity between PAS versus GMS. To evaluate the efficacy of the GMS stain, the investigators identified 326 PAS-negative nail plates submitted for evaluation of possible onychomycosis, which were then stained with GMS. Staining of additional levels with GMS highlighted fungal hyphae in 14 (4.3%) of the 326 PAS-negative nail plate specimens, whereas 312 specimens remained negative.

As a control, the investigators identified 190 additional nail plates negative for PAS on the first level and evaluated a deeper section by a second PAS stain. In this group, 8 (4.2%) revealed fungal hyphae by this methodology. Although the rate of positive staining was not statistically different (4.2% vs 4.3%; $P = .57$), PAS was 2.6-fold less expensive.

Taken together, the investigators conclude that the PAS stain is the optimal method for diagnosing onychomycosis.[12]

A recent study by Idriss and colleagues[13] showed fungal fluorescence of routinely stained sections as a useful diagnostic tool in the diagnosis of onychomycosis. Forty-six of 48 routinely stained PAS-positive onychomycosis nail plate specimens showed positive fluorescence, whereas 20 of 23 PAS-negative control specimens remained negative on fluorescent examination. The sensitivity and specificity of the method were 96% and 90%, respectively. The investigators commented that fungal fluorescence has several distinct advantages, such as no delay associated with a special stain, cheaper cost compared with

PAS, and that it can be performed when tissue is exhausted and not available for special stains.

ONYCHOMYCOSIS

Onychomycosis is the most common disease of the nail unit in adults, presenting with yellow patches and streaks, onycholysis, and subungual hyperkeratosis (**Fig. 2**A).[14] Approximately 75% of onychomycosis is caused by dermatophytes, including *Trichophyton rubrum*, *Trichophyton mentagrophytes*, and *Epidermophyton floccosum*; however, 5% to 15% can be caused by nondermatophyte fungi, such as *Aspergillus*, *Scopulariopsis brevicaulis*, *Scytalidium dimidiatum*, and *Fusarium*.[9,10] Many practitioners empirically treat nail dystrophy as onychomycosis, believing a clinical examination is sufficient for diagnosis and treatment. However, this practice may lead to expensive, ineffective treatment, and drug-related risk exposure without definitive diagnosis of onychomycosis. The American Academy of Dermatology's contribution to the Choosing Wisely campaign specifically highlights clinical similarities between onychomycosis and other nail dermatoses, and urges clinicians not to prescribe oral antifungal therapy for suspected onychomycosis without confirmation of the diagnosis, in order not to subject patients to the risk of unnecessary drug side effects and to avoid inappropriate treatment of the underlying disorder.

Although there are several methods for diagnosis of onychomycosis, such as fungal culture and direct microscopy with KOH, nail clipping for histology with PAS can be particularly helpful. In a recent study by Wilsmann-Theis and colleagues[15] that included 631 samples of onychomycosis shown by at least 1 method, PAS staining of a nail clipping had a higher sensitivity (82%) compared with culture (53%) and direct microscopy (48%). The combination of fungal culture and nail clipping for PAS yielded a sensitivity of 96%, which was higher than combinations of other methods explored in the study.

The advantage of mycologic culture is that it does not only allow the identification of specific fungal species. However, this test is highly operator dependent and therefore less sensitive, at only 35% to 53%.[16] In addition, cultures require long incubation times and can take 4 weeks to

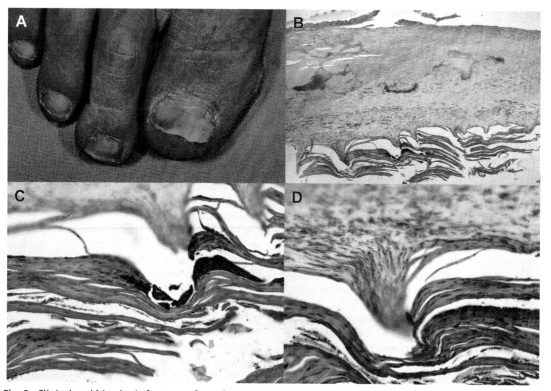

Fig. 2. Clinical and histologic features of onychomycosis. (*A*) The great toenail shows xanthonychia and onycholysis. (*B*) At low power, the nail plate shows thickening and has subungual debris (H&E, 40×). (*C*) At medium power, the nail plate shows parakeratosis, bacteria, and neutrophils at the ventral aspect of the nail plate (H&E, 200×). (*D*) High-power view of the nail plate shows many hyphal elements within the nail plate (PAS, 200×).

return a diagnosis, whereas a nail clipping has a faster turnaround of 2 to 7 days, depending on the laboratory and the complexity of the specimen.

Histopathologic examination of a nail clipping is the least likely modality to be affected by sampling methods or operator experience. Although it is possible to examine the morphology of pathogens with this method, thereby narrowing the differential diagnosis, histologic evaluation of nail clippings cannot precisely identify pathogens and their susceptibilities, or whether the organisms were viable at the time of sampling. It is the most sensitive test to assess for residual infection after therapy with oral antifungal medication.[15] In addition, another disadvantage of obtaining nail clipping for histology is cost, because this method is more expensive than culture and/or direct microscopy.

A nail clipping is also helpful in identifying cases of onychomycosis caused by nondermatophyte fungal infection or coinfection with dermatophyte and nondermatophyte fungi.[17] Several nondermatophyte fungi are resistant to standard antifungal therapies, and therefore culture is necessary to guide therapy. In these cases, the nondermatophyte hyphae may be identified in the nail plate on histologic examination, whereas mycologic culture may be negative.[18] Culture plates use Sabouraud dextrose agar and may contain antibiotics such as cycloheximide that are used to suppress contaminants such as nondermatophyte fungi.[2] Therefore, these hyphae are visible with a PAS examination of the nail plate, but may not grow in culture. The identification of fungal elements within the parenchyma of the nail plate on histologic evaluation in combination with a negative fungal culture from the same nail can therefore raise the possibility of a nondermatophyte onychomycosis.

In addition, nondermatophyte fungi can mask the presence of dermatophytes. Stefanato and Verdolini[18] reported a case of onychomycosis caused by S brevicaulis disguising a dermatophyte infection. Both fungal forms were evident on histologic sections of subungual hyperkeratosis. Culture was only positive for S brevicaulis and repeatedly negative for dermatophyte fungi. On histologic examination, the two fungi maintained separate boundaries, causing territorial demarcation between the infected regions.[18]

Another important histologic phenomenon that may be gleaned from histologic examination of a nail clipping of onychomycosis is the presence of a dermatophytoma.[19] Clinically, a dermatophytoma can present as a round yellow or white patch in the nail plate. A study by Martinez-Herrera and colleagues[20] reported 7 cases of dermatophytoma that clinically presented with white or yellow nail bands with hyperkeratosis, with 3 patients having

total dystrophic onychomycosis, 3 with distal subungual onychomycosis and 1 with superficial white onychomycosis. Microscopic examination of a dermatophytoma shows a dense mass of dermatophyte hyphae.[21] Approximately 18% of patients with onychomycosis present with clinical findings suggesting a dermatophytoma.[19] This presentation is associated with a failure to achieve a mycologic cure following oral antifungal treatment, and treatment with chemical or physical debridement in combination with oral antifungal therapy is recommended. Burkhart and colleagues[22] introduced the concept of biofilm in dermatophyte infections, describing populations or communities of microorganisms that adhere to surfaces and then aggregate, forming a mass or fungal ball because of an extracellular polysaccharide. The biofilm may account for the observed poor therapeutic response and recurrence in the treatment of onychomycosis. Recognizing dermatophytoma on histology and reporting it to the clinician can therefore help guide management and lead to a greater chance of mycologic cure.[19]

The characteristic histologic features in evaluation of onychomycosis are subungual hyperkeratosis, neutrophilic infiltrate, parakeratosis, hemorrhage, and serum crusts (see **Fig. 2**B, C).[23] Most commonly the fungi are located in the ventral aspect of the nail plate. The fungal hyphae on routinely stained sections are difficult to visualize, and are best visualized with PAS or GMS staining. The use of the PAS or GMS stain is essential because there are many overlapping features of onychomycosis and nail unit psoriasis, and it is the presence of hyphae that is the defining feature of onychomycosis (see **Fig. 2**D).[24]

NAIL UNIT PSORIASIS

The characteristic clinical features of psoriasis of the nail are pitting, salmon patches, subungual hyperkeratosis, onycholysis, and splinter hemorrhages (**Fig. 3**A).[25] These changes may be more pronounced in patients with psoriatic arthritis, and some investigators have postulated that the nail changes manifest the extension of the profound inflammation of the distal interphalangeal extensor tendon to involve the nail bed.[26]

However, establishing a diagnosis may be challenging because the clinical features of nail unit psoriasis often overlap with onychomycosis. A nail clipping can be useful in differentiating the two entities by excluding the presence of onychomycosis in patients suspected of having nail psoriasis. The histologic features consistent with psoriasis are a thickened nail plate, subungual

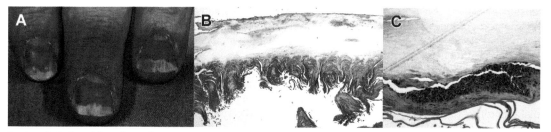

Fig. 3. Clinical and histologic features of nail unit psoriasis. (*A*) Multiple fingernails show onycholysis, oil spots, splinter hemorrhages, and pits. (*B*) Low-power view of nail unit psoriasis shows a thickened nail plate and subungual hyperkeratosis (H&E, 20×). (*C*) High-power view of the nail plate shows areas of parakeratosis with neutrophils within them (H&E, 200×). A PAS stain was negative (not shown).

hyperkeratosis, and parakeratosis, as seen in onychomycosis (see **Fig. 3**B, C).[4,24] The key feature allowing differentiation of nail unit psoriasis and onychomycosis is the lack of fungal elements in psoriasis specimens. However, nail psoriasis is a risk factor for onychomycosis and presence of onychomycosis does not exclude concomitant psoriasis. A nail unit biopsy that includes soft tissue can provide further information to firmly establish a diagnosis of psoriasis.

ONYCHOMATRICOMA

OM is a benign nail unit tumor clinically characterized by a thickened, yellowed, overcurved nail plate with splinter hemorrhages (**Fig. 4**A).[27] OM

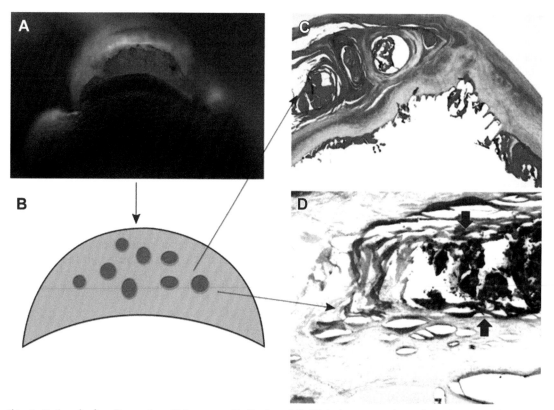

Fig. 4. Rationale for diagnosing OM on a nail clipping. (*A*) Clinical presentation of the honeycomb cavities evident at the frontal margin of the thickened nail plate. (*B*) The nail clipping specimen used for histologic analysis and containing the honeycomb cavities in a thickened, overcurved yellow nail. (*C*) Transverse section shows increased nail thickness with cavitations filled with serous material and surrounded by a layer of epithelium (Hematoxylin-eosin; original magnification ×4). (*D*) Epithelium matrix of the tumor projections indicated by arrows (anticytokeratin antibody; original magnification, 40×). (*From* Miteva M, de Farias DC, Zaiac M, et al. Nail clipping diagnosis of onychomatricoma. Arch Dermatol 2011;147(9):1117; with permission.)

causes a classic honeycomb appearance in the free edge of the nail plate when viewed from the front.[28] This honeycomb appearance is caused by longitudinal tunnels that run the length of the nail plate (see **Fig. 4**B). The clinical presentation of OM is varied and includes a verrucous band pattern suggestive of subungual Bowen disease, total dystrophy of the nail resembling cutaneous horn-type squamous cell carcinoma, and a pseudofibrokeratoma type.[29] OM can also present with dorsal pterygium and longitudinal melanonychia.[29,30] MRI of OM reveals a pathognomonic Y-shaped appearance of the proximal nail plate longitudinally with holes apparent in the transverse plane.[31]

On histology, OM is a biphasic tumor with multiple fibrous projections lined by matrix epithelium, which generates the thickened nail plate.[2] The projections interdigitate into the nail plate causing cleftlike spaces. The cleftlike spaces cause a characteristic honeycomb clinical appearance of the distal thickened nail plate.[32] The fibrous stroma is often organized into 2 layers, with the superficial layer composed of thin wavy fibroblast nuclei oriented in a random array, and the deep layer composed of thick bundles of collagen aligned in a horizontal plane.

Miteva and colleagues[33] recently showed that OM can be diagnosed with the use of a nail clipping. H&E stains of the nail plate sectioned in the transverse plane revealed lacunar spaces, and some were filled with serous debris and lined with matrix epithelium. A pancytokeratin stain was used to highlight the epithelium (see **Fig. 4**C, D). OM seems to be the only nail unit tumor to cause this histologic appearance within the nail plate. Use of a nail clipping to diagnose OM can help with patient diagnosis as well as surgical planning if the tumor goes on to be excised. The diagnosis can be confirmed by excision of the tumor. This noninvasive technique of diagnosis by nail clipping can provide the diagnosis of a benign growth and spare the patient potential morbidity from an excisional procedure.[33]

SUBUNGUAL HEMATOMA

Nail pigmentation is often a cause for concern for neoplastic processes, including malignant melanoma, but is also seen in the setting of trauma leading to subungual hemorrhage. A nail clipping can aid in identifying subungual hematoma, particularly when the lesion is at the distal aspect of the nail plate. If subungual hematoma is confirmed, it may spare the patient from undergoing a more extensive nail unit biopsy, which carries higher morbidity and greater risk of complications. However, clinicians must be cautious when attributing nail pigmentation to subungual hemorrhage alone and ensure clinical resolution of the lesion, because the observed bleeding may be caused by an underlying neoplasm.

Histologic identification of subungual hematoma requires an area of collection of blood within, or clearly associated with, the nail plate (**Fig. 5**). A diaminobenzidine stain can be used to confirm and identify an area of hemorrhage, and can be particularly helpful in clippings with only a focal area of hemorrhage present.

NAIL CLIPPING FOR NAIL UNIT BIOPSY PLANNING OF MELANONYCHIA

Melanonychia is a common chief complaint in the nail clinic, with a broad differential diagnosis (**Fig. 6**A). Nonneoplastic causes in the differential diagnosis of melanonychia include subungual hematoma, infections, foreign material, drugs, Laugier-Hunziker syndrome, Peutz-Jeghers syndrome, nutritional deficiency, ethnic nail pigmentation, and postinflammatory hyperpigmentation.[34] Neoplastic causes include subungual

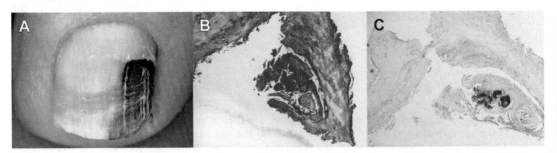

Fig. 5. Clinical and histologic features of a subungual hematoma. (*A*) Clinical presentation shows pigmentation at the medial aspect of the nail with clear nail plate at the proximal aspect. (*B*) Medium-power view shows the nail plate associated with a collection of hemorrhage (H&E, 100×). (*C*) Diaminobenzidine staining highlights the collection of blood (diaminobenzidine, 100×).

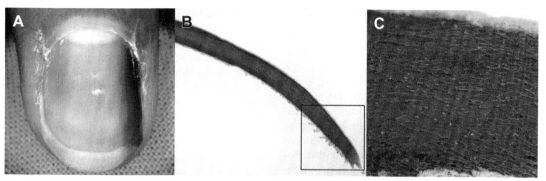

Fig. 6. Nail clipping of melanonychia. (*A*) There is longitudinal melanonychia on a single nail unit. (*B*) Fontana staining of a nail clipping is shown at low power. The box corresponds with the area magnified in *C* (Fontana, 20×). (*C*) High-power view of Fontana-stained sections shows pigmentation throughout all layers of the nail plate, and this predicts that the lesion extends through the proximal and distal matrix (Fontana, 200×).

pigmented Bowen disease, pigmented squamous cell carcinoma, and melanocytic proliferations such as lentigines, melanocytic nevi, and melanoma.[34] Given concern for neoplasia, a soft tissue biopsy is often necessary to establish a definitive diagnosis. However, this often raises the concern for a permanent postprocedure nail dystrophy.

A nail clipping can be a useful adjunct to aid in the surgical planning, to predict the area of the nail matrix from which a pigmented lesion arises. Having this information helps plan the surgical approach, and is useful in counseling patients on the likelihood and severity of postprocedure permanent nail dystrophy. The dorsal aspect of the nail plate is created by the proximal matrix, whereas the ventral aspect of the nail plate is created by distal matrix. Nail surgery in the proximal matrix has a high risk for permanent nail dystrophy, whereas the risk in the distal portion is lower. By clipping and examining the distribution of the pigment clinicians can predict the anatomic areas of the matrix that are affected, and plan and counsel the patient accordingly.

On histology, this is accomplished with the use of Fontana staining (see **Fig. 6**B, C), which highlights the melanin pigmentation and its distribution within the nail plate. Pigmentation in the dorsal aspect of the nail plate predicts a lesion located in the proximal matrix, whereas pigmentation localized to the ventral aspect of the nail plate predicts a lesion located in the distal matrix. If the entire thickness of the nail plate contains pigment, this predicts a lesion that extends throughout the proximal and distal matrix. Not only does use of a nail clipping facilitate surgical planning, but this maneuver helps to exclude a pigmented onychomycosis as the cause of the melanonychia.

PIGMENTED ONYCHOMYCOSIS

The differential diagnosis for melanonychia includes pigmented onychomycosis, which can be identified on histologic evaluation of a nail clipping. Although most onychomycosis is caused by infection with dermatophytes, the incidence of onychomycosis caused by nondermatophytic molds such as dematiaceous fungi, which are notoriously difficult to treat, is increasing. The dematiaceous fungus *Scytalidium dimidiatum* and the nondematiaceous dermatophyte *T rubrum* are the most frequently isolated agents of fungal melanonychia, followed by dematiaceous fungi of the genera *Alternaria* and *Exophiala*.[35] These organisms produce melanin, which is incorporated into their cell walls or secreted extracellularly, causing them to appear brown to black when cultured. Pigmented onychomycosis can diffusely affect the entire nail or present as a longitudinal band, mimicking a pigmented lesion. A clinical clue to distinguish these two entities is that pigmented onychomycosis often spares the matrix, whereas a pigmented lesion most commonly originates in the matrix.

Histology of pigmented onychomycosis is characterized by nail plate thickening, subungual hyperkeratosis, and parakeratosis as in all cases of onychomycosis; however, no special stains are needed for the diagnosis of pigmented onychomycosis, because the hyphae are pigmented and easily visualized on routinely prepared sections.

It is important to keep in mind that nail clipping, although useful for some diagnoses, is not exhaustive, and onychomycosis may coexist with other inflammatory dermatoses affecting the nail unit, as well as malignancies. This point needs to be considered in patients not responding to antifungal therapy for pigmented onychomycosis.

NAIL COSMETICS

Cosmetic enhancement of the nail unit is a popular practice and constitutes a multibillion dollar industry in the United States.[36] However, the presence or absence of nail cosmetics adherent to a nail plate specimen is rarely specified by the submitting clinician. It is important to be aware of the histologic features of nail cosmetics because they have the potential to be confused with disorders affecting the nail unit, in particular subungual hematoma, dyschromias, and other foreign materials.[37] Recognition of the histologic features can thus decrease unnecessary and costly work-ups. Our group previously reported multiple histologic patterns of nail unit cosmetics. These patterns include linear hyperpigmentation with diffuse fine granular material and no apparent polarizable material, linear layered material with a single linear band of polarizable material, and linear hyperpigmentation with larger granules and crystals of polarizable material. A clue that material identified may be a nail cosmetic is that nail cosmetics are found on the dorsal aspect of the nail plate on a nail clipping specimen (**Fig. 7**).

FORENSIC APPLICATIONS OF NAIL CLIPPINGS

Fingernail scrapings and clippings are routinely examined in forensic casework if the case history suggests their evidentiary relevance. DNA extracted from fingernail clippings of victims in forensic cases in which victims struggled or defended themselves is a possible source of DNA from the perpetrator.[38] The DNA on a victim's fingernails could possibly originate from contact with the suspect's blood, saliva, semen, or scratched skin.[39] However, findings from DNA typing from forensic cases of nail clippings are often low yield, because of small sample size and the need for rapid sample recovery and processing, which is often not possible.[40] Matte and colleagues[41] conducted several controlled studies examining the incidence of foreign DNA profiles beneath fingernails and its utility in forensic analysis. In their analysis of forensic casework data (n = 265), 33% of fingernail samples revealed a foreign source of DNA. In a sampling of fingernails from the general population (n = 178), 19% contained a foreign source of DNA. In a study involving deliberate scratching of another individual (n = 30), 33% of individuals had a foreign DNA profile beneath their fingernails from which the person they scratched could not be excluded as the source; however, when sampling occurred approximately 6 hours after the scratching event, only 7% retained the foreign DNA. The investigators concluded that their studies suggest that the incidence of foreign DNA profiles beneath fingernails in the general population is low but, when present, most are of limited significance and tend not to persist for an extensive period of time.

Another application of nail clipping in forensics is in evaluation for exposure to heavy metals, such as arsenic. Arsenic in drinking water is thought to be an environmental toxin and carcinogen.[42] Arsenic has historically been deliberately used as a poison because of its nearly tasteless and odorless qualities. Symptoms of acute arsenic poisoning are numerous and include nausea, emesis, abdominal pain, rice-water diarrhea, hepatitis, pancytopenia, anemia, basophilic stippling arrhythmias, encephalopathy, polyneuropathy, renal insufficiency, or renal failure.[43] With chronic exposure,

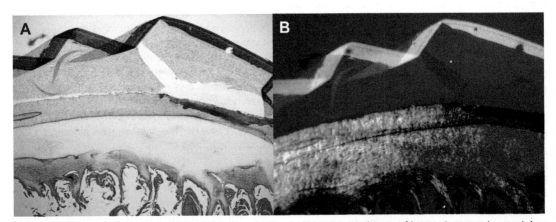

Fig. 7. Nail clipping with nail cosmetics. (*A*) Nail cosmetics can be seen as 2 layers of hyperpigmented material on the dorsal aspect of the nail plate (H&E, 40×). (*B*) The top layer of nail cosmetic is highlighted with polarization (H&E, 40×; polarized microscopy).

dermatologic changes including Mees lines, arsenical keratosis, generalized hyperpigmentation, or alopecia, as well as systemic damage such as cirrhosis, hypertension, peripheral vascular disease, stocking glove neuropathy, tremor, or malignancies, may be seen.[44] An increase in the incidence of skin, bladder, and lung cancers at high arsenic concentrations is well established.[45] In the United States, an estimated 13 million people are exposed to arsenic concentrations that exceed the US Environmental Protection Agency's maximum contaminant level.[46]

Because of the short half-life of arsenic in the blood, urine is the preferred specimen for detection of acute exposure. Trivalent inorganic arsenic binds to the sulfhydryl groups in nail onychocytes and thus makes toenail arsenic a good measure of chronic or past (>3 weeks) arsenic exposure.[42] Depending on the speed of nail growth, toenail measurements represent exposures that occurred 1 to 12 months before sample collection.

Nail clipping samples requiring heavy metal testing can be sent to reference laboratories for analysis. Quantitative inductively coupled plasma/mass spectrometry assays for a variety of metals, including arsenic, lead, mercury, and thallium, are available. For patients undergoing evaluation, nail samples of at least 500 mg are required, and should be packaged separately in an acid-washed or trace metal–free plastic container. For postmortem cases, the entire nail should be submitted, with individual nails packaged separately in individual plastic bottles or bags.

DRUGS IN NAILS

Nail clippings can also be used to identify the presence of orally ingested prescription medications as well as illicit drug exposure. Although methodologies using body fluids such as serum or urine are used in analysis of short-term exposures, nail clippings have the advantage of providing information regarding retrospective drug exposure. Drugs are incorporated into the nail plate by a double mechanism of deposition into the root of the nail via blood flow into the nail matrix, as well as transfer from the nail bed during growth from the lunula to the beginning of the free margin.[47] Among prescription medications that can be analyzed from a nail clipping are antifungal medications, which in studies allow target concentration monitoring and the determination of onychomycosis treatment periods. Determining the optimal treatment period can help reduce adverse effects. Other prescription medications that can be analyzed from a nail clipping are neuroleptics, anticonvulsants, and the antiviral agent indinavir,[48] allowing assessment of medication compliance. Long-term retention in the nails of numerous illicit substances, including amphetamines, cannabinoids, cocaine, benzodiazepines, and opioids, can be used for detection of drug abuse.[47,48] In addition, nail clippings may be used for assessment of intrauterine exposure to drugs that may be suspected to have caused fetal damage or congenital abnormalities.

Table 1	
Optimization for collection and interpretation of nail clippings	
Procedural Aspect	**Optimization**
Instruments	Double-action nail nipper or heavy-duty nail clipper for thick nails
Sufficient sample	Free edge of nail plate should be at least 4 mm. If not sufficient, patient should return
Anatomic area for nail clipping	Clip as proximal as possible without causing pain; also include subungual hyperkeratosis
Pathology requisition	Clearly indicate that a nail clipping is present and any special requests or clinical concerns
Grossing	Use a softening solution to aid in ease of cutting tissue
Microtomy	Blocks can be partially immersed in a softening solution to aid in passing of blade to enhance tissue section quality
Tissue adherence to slide	Use adhesive to ensure good contact between slide and tissue sections. Place slides for 1 h in a 65°–75°C oven to ensure that the nail sections adhere to the slide before staining
Fungal stains	Literature at this time favors PAS rather than GMS for efficiency and cost savings
Specimen interpretation	Consider immunofluorescence microscopy if tissue is exhausted before preparation of fungal stains

Table 2
Clinical and nail clipping histopathologic features of common nail unit dermatoses

Diagnosis	Clinical Features	Nail Clipping Histology
Onychomycosis	Nail plate thickening, xanthonychia, onycholysis, subungual hyperkeratosis	Hyperkeratosis, neutrophils, parakeratosis, plasma globules, and fungal elements
Dermatophytoma	Leukonychia or xanthonychia arranged as a linear spike or circular area in the nail plate	Compact mass of fungal elements within and associated with the nail plate
Nail unit psoriasis	Nail plate thickening, oil spots, pitting, onycholysis, subungual hyperkeratosis, splinter hemorrhages	Hyperkeratosis, neutrophils, parakeratosis
Onychomatricoma	Overcurved nail plate with xanthonychia, splinter hemorrhages, and a honeycomb appearance when viewed from front	Multiple circular channels that may have cytokeratin-positive associated epithelium
Subungual hematoma	Irregular nail pigmentation usually not continuous with the proximal nail fold	Nail plate–associated hemorrhage, which can be highlighted with diaminobenzidine staining

SUMMARY

This article summarizes the practical approach (**Table 1**), utility, and histologic findings of nail clippings in evaluation of onychomycosis, nail unit psoriasis, OM, melanonychia, subungual hematoma, and nail cosmetics, as well as the forensic applications of this easily obtained specimen (**Table 2**). This summary is intended to enable dermatologists to expand their use of this everyday procedure to enhance their ability to diagnose dermatoses affecting the nail unit.

REFERENCES

1. Kovich OI, Soldano AC. Clinical pathologic correlations for diagnosis and treatment of nail disorders. Dermatol Ther 2007;20(1):11–6.
2. Stewart CL, Rubin AI. Update: nail unit dermatopathology. Dermatol Ther 2012;25(6):551–68.
3. Suarez SM, Silvers DN, Scher RK, et al. Histologic evaluation of nail clippings for diagnosing onychomycosis. Arch Dermatol 1991;127(10):1517–9.
4. André J, Sass U, Richert B, et al. Nail pathology. Clin Dermatol 2013;31(5):526–39.
5. Lewin K, DeWit SA, Lawson R. Softening techniques for nail biopsies. Arch Dermatol 1973; 107(2):223–4.
6. Orchard GE, Torres J, Southhararajah R. Use of softening agents to improve the production of formalin-fixed, paraffin-embedded sections of nail tissue: an assessment. Br J Biomed Sci 2008;65(2):68–70.
7. Nazarian RM, Due B, Deshpande A, et al. An improved method of surgical pathology testing for onychomycosis. J Am Acad Dermatol 2012;66(4): 655–60.
8. Chang A, Wharton J, Tam S, et al. A modified approach to the histologic diagnosis of onychomycosis. J Am Acad Dermatol 2007;57(5):849–53.
9. D'Hue Z, Perkins SM, Billings SD. GMS is superior to PAS for diagnosis of onychomycosis. J Cutan Pathol 2008;35(8):745–7.
10. Reza Kermanshahi T, Rhatigan R. Comparison between PAS and GMS stains for the diagnosis of onychomycosis. J Cutan Pathol 2010;37(10):1041–4.
11. Mayer E, Izhak OB, Bergman R. Histopathological periodic acid-Schiff stains of nail clippings as a second-line diagnostic tool in onychomycosis. Am J Dermatopathol 2012;34(3):270–3.
12. Barak O, Asarch A, Horn T. PAS is optimal for diagnosing onychomycosis. J Cutan Pathol 2010;37(10): 1038–40.
13. Idriss MH, Khalil A, Elston D. The diagnostic value of fungal fluorescence in onychomycosis. J Cutan Pathol 2013;40(4):385–90.
14. Effendy I, Lecha M, Feuilhade de Chauvin M, et al, European Onychomycosis Observatory. Epidemiology and clinical classification of onychomycosis. J Eur Acad Dermatol Venereol 2005; 19(Suppl 1):8–12.
15. Wilsmann-Theis D, Sareika F, Bieber T, et al. New reasons for histopathological nail-clipping examination in the diagnosis of onychomycosis. J Eur Acad Dermatol Venereol 2011;25(2):235–7.
16. Karimzadegan-Nia M, Mir-Amin-Mohammadi A, Bouzari N, et al. Comparison of direct smear, culture and histology for the diagnosis of onychomycosis. Australas J Dermatol 2007;48(1):18–21.

17. Pierard GE, Quatresooz P, Arrese JE. Spotlight on nail histomycology. Dermatol Clin 2006;24(3):371–4.

18. Stefanato CM, Verdolini R. Histopathologic evidence of the nondermatophytic mould scopulariopsis *brevicaulis* masking the presence of dermatophytes in a toenail infection. J Cutan Pathol 2009;36(Suppl 1):8–12.

19. Bennett D, Rubin AI. Dermatophytoma: a clinicopathologic entity important for dermatologists and dermatopathologists to identify. Int J Dermatol 2013;52(10):1285–7.

20. Martinez-Herrera E, Moreno-Coutino G, Fernandez-Martinez RF, et al. Dermatophytoma: description of 7 cases. J Am Acad Dermatol 2012;66(6):1014–6.

21. Carney C, Tosti A, Daniel R, et al. A new classification system for grading the severity of onychomycosis: onychomycosis severity index. Arch Dermatol 2011;147(11):1277–82.

22. Burkhart CN, Burkhart CG, Gupta AK. Dermatophytoma: recalcitrance to treatment because of existence of fungal biofilm. J Am Acad Dermatol 2002;47(4):629–31.

23. Grover C, Reddy BS, Chaturvedi KU. Onychomycosis and the diagnostic significance of nail biopsy. J Dermatol 2003;30(2):116–22.

24. Martin B. Nail histopathology. Actas Dermosifiliogr 2013;104(7):564–78.

25. Farber EM, Nall L. Nail psoriasis. Cutis 1992;50(3):174–8.

26. Tan AL, Benjamin M, Toumi H, et al. The relationship between the extensor tendon enthesis and the nail in distal interphalangeal joint disease in psoriatic arthritis–a high-resolution MRI and histological study. Rheumatology (Oxford) 2007;46(2):253–6.

27. Cloetingh D, Helm KF, Ioffreda MD, et al. JAAD grand rounds quiz. onychomatricoma. J Am Acad Dermatol 2014;70(2):395–7.

28. Sanchez M, Hu S, Miteva M, et al. Onychomatricoma has channel-like structures on in vivo reflectance confocal microscopy. J Eur Acad Dermatol Venereol 2014;28(11):1560–2.

29. Perrin C, Baran R, Balaguer T, et al. Onychomatricoma: new clinical and histological features. A review of 19 tumors. Am J Dermatopathol 2010;32(1):1–8.

30. Lam C, Weyant GW, Billingsley EM. Longitudinal melanonychia of the toenail. JAMA Dermatol 2014;150(4):449–50.

31. Perrin C, Baran R. Onychomatricoma with dorsal pterygium: pathogenic mechanisms in 3 cases. J Am Acad Dermatol 2008;59(6):990–4.

32. Perrin C, Langbein L, Schweizer J, et al. Onychomatricoma in the light of the microanatomy of the normal nail unit. Am J Dermatopathol 2011;33(2):131–9.

33. Miteva M, de Farias DC, Zaiac M, et al. Nail clipping diagnosis of onychomatricoma. Arch Dermatol 2011;147(9):1117–8.

34. Amin B, Nehal KS, Jungbluth AA, et al. Histologic distinction between subungual lentigo and melanoma. Am J Surg Pathol 2008;32(6):835–43.

35. Finch J, Arenas R, Baran R. Fungal melanonychia. J Am Acad Dermatol 2012;66(5):830–41.

36. Chang RM, Hare AQ, Rich P. Treating cosmetically induced nail problems. Dermatol Ther 2007;20(1):54–9.

37. Anolik RB, Elenitsas R, Minakawa S, et al. Histologic features of nail cosmetics. Am J Dermatopathol 2012;34(4):412–5.

38. Anderson TD, Ross JP, Roby RK, et al. A validation study for the extraction and analysis of DNA from human nail material and its application to forensic casework. J Forensic Sci 1999;44(5):1053–6.

39. Wiegand P, Bajanowski T, Brinkmann B. DNA typing of debris from fingernails. Int J Legal Med 1993;106(2):81–3.

40. Oz C, Zamir A. An evaluation of the relevance of routine DNA typing of fingernail clippings for forensic casework. J Forensic Sci 2000;45(1):158–60.

41. Matte M, Williams L, Frappier R, et al. Prevalence and persistence of foreign DNA beneath fingernails. Forensic Sci Int Genet 2012;6(2):236–43.

42. Heck JE, Andrew AS, Onega T, et al. Lung cancer in a U.S. population with low to moderate arsenic exposure. Environ Health Perspect 2009;117(11):1718–23.

43. Rusyniak DE, Arroyo A, Acciani J, et al. Heavy metal poisoning: management of intoxication and antidotes. EXS 2010;100:365–96.

44. Singh N, Kumar D, Sahu AP. Arsenic in the environment: effects on human health and possible prevention. J Environ Biol 2007;28(2 Suppl):359–65.

45. Cohen SM, Arnold LL, Beck BD, et al. Evaluation of the carcinogenicity of inorganic arsenic. Crit Rev Toxicol 2013;43(9):711–52.

46. US EPA (US Environmental Protection Agency). National primary drinking water regulations; arsenic and clarifications to compliance and new source contaminants monitoring; final rule. Fed Reg 2001;66:6975–7066.

47. Daniel CR 3rd, Piraccini BM, Tosti A. The nail and hair in forensic science. J Am Acad Dermatol 2004;50(2):258–61.

48. Palmeri A, Pichini S, Pacifici R, et al. Drugs in nails: physiology, pharmacokinetics and forensic toxicology. Clin Pharmacokinet 2000;38(2):95–110.

How to Submit a Nail Specimen

Erica Reinig, MD[a], Phoebe Rich, MD[b], Curtis T. Thompson, MD[a,b,c],*

KEYWORDS

- Biopsy • Microscopy • Histology • Tissue • Sectioning • Orientation • Cassette • Formalin

KEY POINTS

- Proper specimen orientation is crucial for accurate grossing as well as proper tissue embedding and sectioning, significantly improving pathologic diagnostic ability.
- Close communication with the laboratory, including a thorough clinical history and differential and instructions to the laboratory (ie, initial level hematoxylin and eosin stain [H&E] sections), is important.
- Submitting nail biopsy specimens with a specific protocol that includes placing the tissue on a drawing of a nail allows for preservation of orientation and prevents loss of tissue.
- A simple protocol on nail plate specimens greatly improves adherence of the plate to the glass slide for H&E and periodic acid–Schiff (PAS) sections.

INTRODUCTION

Laboratory technicians and pathologists often fear receiving a nail unit specimen because there are significant challenges in both getting the nail plate to adhere to a glass slide and because the soft tissue specimens of the nail unit matrix and bed are often small and fragmented. Interpretation by the pathologist is challenging, not only because of the often difficult nature of the specimen but also because orientation at the microscopic level is tricky, especially when examining a diseased nail unit.

When routine skin specimens are obtained in a clinic, the specimens are usually placed free floating in a container with an appropriate amount of formalin (10% formaldehyde) before the specimen is sent to the laboratory. With nail unit specimens, however, placing these specimens free in formaldehyde results in loss of orientation and frequent loss of critical tissue needed to make a diagnosis. Maintenance of tissue integrity and orientation streamlines specimen processing—from grossing to embedding to sectioning—and significantly improves pathologic diagnostic ability. Thus, in the clinic, nail unit specimens require additional work to preserve tissue integrity and orientation.

It is helpful to be able to send nail unit specimens to a laboratory with expertise in nail specimen processing. However, the clinic is often required to send to a variety of laboratories. By preparing a nail unit specimen in the clinic in a way that preserves orientation and prevents loss of tissue, the specimen may thus be processed and interpreted in a variety of laboratories with better success. Thus, the onus is on the clinician and the clinic to submit nail specimens in a manner as discussed later.

Clear communication with the laboratory is important in nail unit specimen submission. Of primary importance is instruction to the laboratory to pay close attention to small fragments of tissue.

Disclosures: None.
[a] Department of Pathology, Oregon Health Sciences University, Portland, OR, USA; [b] Department of Dermatology, Oregon Health Sciences University, Portland, OR, USA; [c] Department of Biomedical Engineering, Oregon Health Sciences University, Portland, OR, USA
* Corresponding author. PO Box 230577, Portland, OR 97281.
E-mail address: cthompson@cta-lab.com

Dermatol Clin 33 (2015) 303–307
http://dx.doi.org/10.1016/j.det.2014.12.012
0733-8635/15/$ – see front matter Published by Elsevier Inc.

Instructions to perform initial level sections and unstained sections on positively charged slides are important because the small nail matrix/bed specimens may not survive refacing the paraffin block for additional sections. Also important is a clear clinical history and differential, especially because the histologic features of some nail tumors such as onychopapilloma are not distinct. A pathologist not given a clear differential will diagnose an onychopapilloma as a verruca, as both have hyperkeratosis and hypergranulosis. Similarly, a diagnosis of a mold infection requires direction by the clinician to the laboratory to consider a mold; otherwise, the microbiology laboratory will consider the mold a contaminant and not characterize the mold.

For submission in a way that preserves specimen orientation, a couple of methods have previously been proposed. George and colleagues[1] describe a technique of marking the epithelial surface with colored ink, dipping the specimen in glacial acetic acid to fix the ink, and then placing it in formalin for transport. Although this technique may certainly improve orientation by maintaining the ability to identify the epithelial surface, placing the specimen floating free in formalin will lead to a loss of proximal-distal and medial-lateral orientation, and small fragments of potentially diagnostic tissue may be lost. Richert and colleagues[2] describe a different technique for submission in which the specimen is placed on cardboard with a nail diagram and covered with a sheet of filter paper. The cardboard and filter paper are then stapled together so that the specimen remains flat and oriented, preventing tissue loss.

A SIMPLE TECHNIQUE FOR SPECIMEN SUBMISSION

The authors have developed a technique that incorporates aspects of both of these methods, but which may be more practical, particularly in clinics where nail unit sampling is not routine. Borrowing from ophthalmologic tissue processing, the specimen is oriented by placing it on a cartoon printout of a nail (Fig. 1) in the same location as its in vivo location. Multiple tissue fragments may be placed on a single nail cartoon in the area from which they came. Any type of paper may be used for the cartoon, and the cartoon may be drawn by hand with a pen or pencil or printed and cut out (a cartoon printout may currently be found at www.cta-lab.com/nail_resources.html). The cartoon should be small enough to fit flat within a tissue cassette. Wetting the paper slightly with formalin before placing the tissue on it prevents histologic drying artifacts in the tissue.

After placing the specimen on the nail cartoon, the orientation may be further improved by carefully inking one or more edges of the specimen and the corresponding cartoon paper (see Fig. 1). Very precise inking is best done using the wooden end of a cotton swab rather than the cotton end (see Fig. 1C). Because many lesions are pigmented, avoiding black ink is important to prevent confusion of ink with melanin. Thus, green or blue ink is best.

The specimen on the cartoon printout is then placed in a tissue cassette. Tissue cassettes and the sponges that go inside them to secure tissue must be purchased in bulk, so requesting a handful of cassettes and sponges from your local histopathology laboratory is best. After placing 1 or 2 tissue sponges over the cartoon holding the tissue, the cassette is closed securely. The cassette can then be placed in an appropriately sized container with formalin for fixation and transportation to the laboratory (Fig. 2).

On receipt in the laboratory, the cassette holding the nail unit specimen may be sent directly through overnight processing without opening the cassette. The tissue may also undergo gross sectioning before overnight processing. Small fragments may move around a little on the cartoon during the overnight processing, but the overnight processing adds significant strength to the soft tissue and often leads to the ability to perform more precise gross sectioning. The histotechnologist should be encouraged to consult the pathologist for advice on orientation, inking, and gross sectioning. For instance, features of a presumed onychopapilloma are best seen with longitudinal proximal-to-distal sections, whereas features of an onychomatricoma are best seen with transverse sections. In addition, a fragmented specimen may be separated by the histotechnologist into multiple separate cassettes or blocks. Finally, the laboratory should be instructed to cut 5 to 10 unstained sections on positively charged slides with the initial hematoxylin and eosin stain (H&E) sections for use with additional H&E or special stains; this prevents loss of potentially critical tissue needed to make an accurate diagnosis.

NAIL PLATE SUBMISSION

Nail plate associated with a matrix/bed specimen should be submitted separately from the soft tissue if possible. This separate submission is because the histotechnologist is often most concerned about sectioning the very hard nail plate, and the diagnostic tissue is usually the matrix/bed specimen. Failure to separate the soft tissue from the plate may result in loss of diagnostic

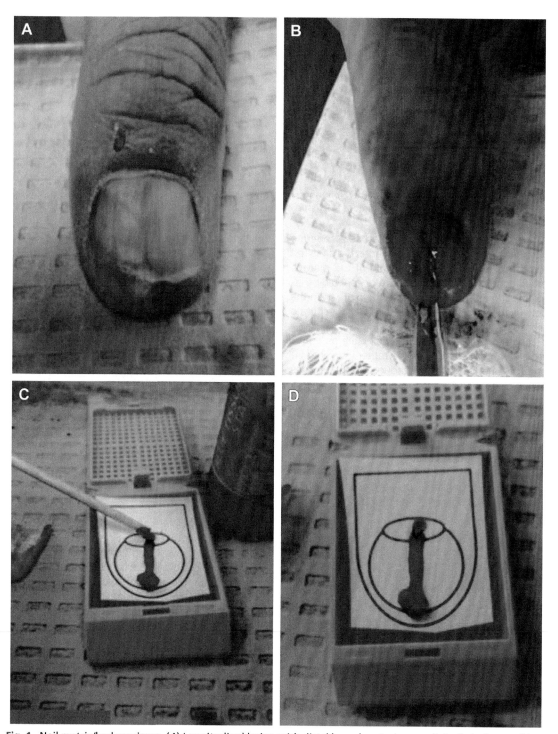

Fig. 1. Nail matrix/bed specimen. (*A*) Longitudinal lesion with distal hyperkeratosis seen clinically before excision. (*B*) Longitudinal lesion in the nail matrix/bed after removal of the nail plate. (*C*) Excised specimen on the nail diagram in the tissue cassette being inked proximally (matrix). (*D*) Excised, inked specimen on the nail diagram in the tissue cassette.

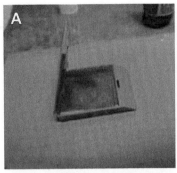
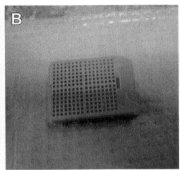
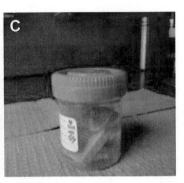

Fig. 2. Tissue cassette holding specimen. (*A*) Sponge over inked specimen on nail diagram in the tissue cassette. (*B*) Close tissue cassette holding specimen. (*C*) Tissue cassette in a container with 10% formalin.

tissue. The plate may be submitted as a separate specimen or in the same container as the cassette to reduce laboratory cost (**Fig. 3**). If the plate is attached to soft tissue, the laboratory should be instructed to attempt to separate the plate from the soft tissue and to process them as a separate blocks or slides.

Many nail surgeons use the nail plate as a protective barrier after the surgery rather than submitting it to the laboratory. Although the plate does not re-adhere to the nail matrix/bed, the natural shape of the plate is quite useful as a protective cover. It remains controversial whether important diagnostic tissue is being lost with this practice, because epithelium may remain attached to the plate after surgical reflection, which may contain diagnostic clues, especially for melanoma.[3] In the authors' experience, proper reflection of the nail plate using a small, thin Freer elevator results

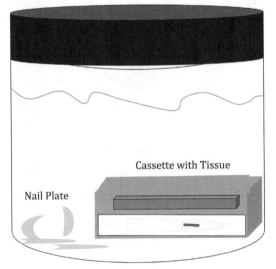

Fig. 3. Nail plate submitted in the same container as a tissue cassette holding the matrix/bed specimen reduces laboratory fees but does not compromise the quality of the specimen.

in almost all of the epithelium remaining in the matrix/bed and not on the plate.[4]

Finally, although onychomycosis may not be the primary disease process, dystrophic nail plate over a lesion is often secondarily infected with fungus, and a periodic acid–Schiff (PAS) stain should always be performed on the plate.

PROTOCOL FOR ADHERENCE OF NAIL PLATE TO A GLASS SLIDE

Successful processing of nail plate so that it remains adhered to the glass slide is a challenge in most laboratories. As such, a plethora of techniques exist to achieve this, most which have not been assessed in a controlled study. Of particular note is the use of the hair removal product, Nair, by many laboratories. Laboratories also coat the slides with a variety of products, such as gelatin. In the authors' experience, gelatin coating significantly improves plate adherence and subsequent staining. Preparation of the slide before PAS staining can be achieved with a high level of success with the preparation detailed in **Box 1**, in which gelatin is added to the water bath, where the tissue floats after sectioning. Of important note, a PAS stain on a slide of nail plate should not undergo diastase treatment, because this causes the plate to come off the glass slide.

SUBMISSION OF NAIL PLATE FOR FUNGUS IDENTIFICATION

Submitting a nail plate and debris for fungus and mold identification is best done by submitting the material dry in a small envelope. The sample may then be prepared for H&E and PAS sections and submitted for culture. Sampling of the nail unit for fungus, including mold, should be directed to the site of suspected infection, because a variety of infectious patterns exist (distal lateral subungual, white superficial, proximal subungual, endonyx, and candidal onychomycosis).[5] Multiple

> **Box 1**
> **Slide preparation of nail plate for periodic acid–Schiff staining**
>
> *Procedure*
> 1. Place a small amount of gelatin in the water bath
> 2. Pick up desired sections using positively charged slides
> 3. Place in oven at 60°C for 30–60 min (increase time for "difficult" specimens)
> 4. Deparaffinize slides using xylene or xylene substitutes
> 5. Hydrate through a series of standard alcohols
> 6. Rinse slide in running cool tap water
> 7. Rinse slide in distilled water
> 8. DO NOT "DIGEST" SLIDES!!!
> 9. Proceed to PAS solution staining using a standard protocol

techniques for sampling exist, including drilling into the nail plate to obtain the sample.[6]

SUBMISSION OF A PIGMENTED BAND SPECIMEN

Because nail unit sampling is often done for a pigmented band and because the histopathologic findings may be quite subtle, it is important to instruct the laboratory on performing up-front special stains as follows:

1. Level H&E sections (3 slides)
2. MelanA (Mart-1) immunohistochemical stain to characterize melanocyte number, size, and density
3. Fontana-Masson stain to identify melanin
4. PAS stain to identify pigmented fungus
5. Five to 10 unstained sections on charged slides for possible additional H&E and special stains.

Blood in the nail unit may also produce pigmentation, often associated with trauma. Blood within the nail plate is almost always visible on an H&E section, and a special stain is not needed. A Perl iron stain will not work, because the iron moiety in the heme has not been released through oxidation if it is in the nail unit. A benzidine stain will identify the blood; however, benzidine is carcinogenic and difficult to use in the laboratory, and, as noted, the erythrocytes are almost always visible on the H&E sections.[7]

SUMMARY

As previously mentioned, given the paucity of specific protocols, many nail biopsies are received fragmented and without orientation. With such specimens, proper grossing, processing, and embedding can be exceedingly difficult. Through careful submission of the specimen as outlined above, more accurate diagnoses are possible.

REFERENCES

1. George R, Clarke S, Ioffreda M, et al. Marking of nail matrix biopsies with ink aids in proper specimen orientation for more accurate histologic evaluation. Dermatol Surg 2008;34(12):1705–6.
2. Richert B, Theunis A, Norrenberg S, et al. Tangential excision of pigmented nail matrix lesions responsible for longitudinal melanonychia: evaluation of the technique on a series of 30 patients. J Am Acad Dermatol 2013;69(1):96–104.
3. Rueben BS, McCalmont TH. The importance of attached nail plate epithelium in the diagnosis of nail apparatus melanoma. J Cutan Pathol 2010; 37(10):1027–9.
4. Daniel CR III. Basic nail plate avulsion. J Dermatol Surg Oncol 1992;18:685–8.
5. Baran R, Hay RJ, Tosti A, et al. A new classification of onychomycosis. Br J Dermatol 1998;139(4):567–71.
6. Shemer A, Trau H, Davidovici B, et al. Collection of fungi samples from nails: comparative study of curettage and drilling techniques. J Eur Acad Dermatol Venereol 2008;22(2):182–5.
7. Rueben BS. Pigmented lesions of the nail unit: clinical and histologic features. Semin Cutan Med Surg 2010; 29:148–58.

Index

Note: Page numbers of article titles are in **boldface** type.

Dermatol Clin 33 (2015) 309–313
http://dx.doi.org/10.1016/S0733-8635(15)00010-8
0733-8635/15/$ – see front matter © 2015 Elsevier Inc. All rights reserved.

derm.theclinics.com

Printed and bound by CPI Group (UK) Ltd, Croydon, CR0 4YY

03/10/2024

01040377-0010